Diagnostic Reasoning in Nursing

Doris L. Carnevali, R.N., M.N.

Associate Professor Emeritus, Community Health Care Systems Department
University of Washington School of Nursing

Pamela H. Mitchell, R.N., C.N.R.N., M.S., F.A.A.N.

Professor, Physiologic Nursing Department
University of Washington School of Nursing
Neurological Nurse Specialist, Division of Neurology–Neurosurgery

Nancy F. Woods, R.N., Ph.D., F.A.A.N.

Professor Physiologic Nursing Department
Director, Office of Nursing Research Facilitation
University of Washington School of Nursing

Christine A. Tanner, R.N., Ph.D.

Associate Professor, Department of Adult Health and Illness
Director, Office of Research Development and Utilization
School of Nursing, The Oregon Health Sciences University

with 4 contributors

Carol G. Blainey, R.N., M.N.

Associate Professor, Physiologic Nursing Department
School of Nursing, University of Washington
Clinician, University of Washington Diabetes Research Center

Nancy S. Konikow, R.N., C.N.R.N., M.N.

Clinical Assistant Professor, Physiologic Nursing Department
University of Washington School of Nursing
Neurological Clinical Nurse Specialist—Neurology–Neurosurgery
University Hospital

Ruth McCorkle, R.N., Ph.D., F.A.A.N.

Associate Professor, Community Health Care Systems Department
School of Nursing, University of Washington
Oncology Clinical Specialist

Gail P. Simmons, R.N., B.S.N.

Nurse Practitioner III
University of Washington Hemodialysis Research Facility

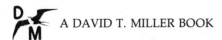 A DAVID T. MILLER BOOK

Diagnostic Reasoning in Nursing

J.B. LIPPINCOTT COMPANY   Philadelphia
London   Mexico City   New York   St. Louis   São Paulo   Sydney

Sponsoring Editor: David T. Miller
Manuscript Editor: Kristen B. Frasch
Indexer: Ellen Murray
Art Director: Tracy Baldwin/Earl Gerhart
Interior Design: Earl Gerhart
Cover Design: Partners Advertising & Design Group
Production Supervisor: J. Corey Gray
Production Assistant: Barney Fernandes
Compositor: Bi-Comp, Incorporated
Printer/Binder: R.R. Donnelley & Sons Company

6 5 4 3 2 1

Library of Congress Cataloging in Publication Data
Main entry under title:

Diagnostic reasoning in nursing.

  Bibliography: p.
  Includes index.
  1. Nursing.   2. Diagnosis.   I. Carnevali, Doris L.
[DNLM: 1. Nursing process. WY 100 D5345]
RT48.D48   1984   616.07'5'0024613   83-16181
ISBN 0-397-54349-2

The authors and publisher have exerted every effort to ensure that drug selection and dosage set forth in this text are in accord with current recommendations and practice at the time of publication. However, in view of ongoing research, changes in government regulations, and the constant flow of information relating to drug therapy and drug reactions, the reader is urged to check the package insert for each drug for any change in indications and dosage and for added warnings and precautions. This is particularly important when the recommended agent is a new or infrequently employed drug.

PREFACE

Two areas important to nursing's continuing development as a health discipline and profession are: 1) the general recognition of nursing's distinctive domain in health care and 2) its clinicians' rigorous, effective and consistent use of the diagnostic reasoning process. Diagnostic Reasoning in Nursing addresses both these areas.

This book describes a relatively concrete and highly pragmatic, field-tested domain for nursing, one that is distinguishable from those of other disciplines. It is subsequently illustrated in four chapters of Section 3, written by practicing clinicians who nurse clientele with varying health problems, nurses who work in both institutional and home-care settings.

The diagnostic reasoning process is described in Chapter 2. This description is then followed by chapters discussing the stages of development of diagnostic reasoning expertise, from novice to expert. The characteristics of diagnostic tasks, the areas of difficulty and constraints, and the strategies used in managing them are identified. The risks to practice associated with each stage of development are also described. In Section 3, the practicing clinicians illustrate how the elements of the diagnostic reasoning process are applied using a purely nursing perspective. The headings in each of the chapters are comparable and serve to illustrate the components of the diagnostic reasoning process. The contributors were asked to assume that the biomedical diagnosing was being competently and concurrently addressed with their clients, so they were to apply the diagnostic reasoning only to the nursing (daily living ↔ health status) perspective.

The fourth section addresses some major professional issues: the issue of taxonomic structure and methods for studying diagnostic reasoning from both process and input–output models. Mathematical models and clinical illustrations are included. The final chapter in this section describes and illustrates the techniques for developing computer-simulation exercises. It also discusses their uses in both teaching and evaluating diagnostic skills.

The fifth and final section addresses implications for various nursing roles once diagnostic reasoning is incorporated as an acknowledged, explicit skill in professional nursing. Concrete strategies for self-analysis and professional growth for the practicing clinician or nursing student are also described. Finally, the implications for a variety of segments of the nursing profession are explored—practice, service, education, literature, and research.

This book can be of use to a wide range of readers. It can serve the needs of students (undergraduate and graduate), teachers, nursing managers, practicing clinicians, nursing researchers, and nursing authors.

Students as well as practicing clinicians can use it as a self-help guide to upgrade their diagnostic skills. It can also be used to test or firm up their working perspective of nursing's territory and perspective.

Nursing educators, with their distinctive difference in perspective from the biomedical orientation, can use the nursing-domain models as a frame of reference for combining *nursing* knowledge and diagnosis *parity* with the biomedical aspects they teach. (This represents a real departure from the consideration of nursing actions as a subset of medical diagnosis and treatment.) This perspective should also enable educators to make clear distinctions when demonstrating how patient data are used differently in nursing and medicine—even the same data. Educators can also use the elements of the diagnostic reasoning process and the stages in development of diagnostic expertise to plan both teaching strategies (in classroom and clinical settings) and evaluation criteria. The constant awareness that nursing students must organize and store knowledge to expedite effective retrieval for diagnostic purposes should influence the organization of material for classroom presentation in lectures and conferences. Modelling parity for nursing and medical diagnosing, both in theory presentations and in clinical practice, can be initiated or enhanced through the use of the case material and ideas presented in the book.

Nursing service managers and administrators can use the ideas in the book for both quality control considerations and for staff development. Content from the book may also be helpful in planning management by objectives, in the nursing diagnostic areas.

Researchers in nursing may see the variables of the models representing the nursing domain, and the diagnostic reasoning components, as conceptual frameworks needed for studies in these areas.

Authors and prospective authors can find this book useful as a frame of reference for organizing the content. They can also use it for perspective, and for the content itself. Nursing literature, most importantly nursing texts that will be used by the next generation of practicing nurses, must seriously consider some basic issues in content and format. These include:

    highlighting and consistently modeling the distinctive
       differences between the nursing and biomedical
       perspectives—in the knowledge that forms nursing's
       foundation, in the data required for a sound data base
       in each domain, and in the focus of diagnosis and
       treatment that each discipline takes,

    modelling appropriate parity and concurrency for
       nursing and biomedical diagnoses and their respective
       distinct treatment regimens, and

    structuring a consistent sequence and format in the
       organization of nursing knowledge (and associated
       biomedical knowledge) to enhance systematic
       organization and storage of that knowledge for
       efficient retrieval in diagnostic reasoning and treatment
       decisions. (See Figure 14-1, page 236 for a sample of
       headings that serves well for both nursing and
       biomedical diagnostic-treatment concepts.)

The nurses who wrote this book will be the first to acknowledge the difficulty of the approach we have taken in thinking and writing—yet the need for nursing literature with this perspective and organization is critical.

    This book limited its scope to the diagnostic reasoning process, using a particular model of the nursing domain. An important area yet to be addressed is the critical thinking process associated with decision making as it applies to treatment options. Also still to be addressed is diagnostic reasoning's critical linkage to a base of knowledge about the underlying mechanisms connecting daily living ↔ health status phenomena that form the rationale for those treatment decisions. This area too needs comparable explicit attention in terms of:

    the process of decision making, as opposed to diagnostic
       thinking,

    substantive content—the "pathology" or underlying
       dynamics of daily living/developmental task
       accomplishments in relation to health status, leading
       to the rationale for treatment options and variants, and

    effective formats for organization and storage of this
       knowledge to expedite sound treatment decisions and
       evaluation.

This demanding task awaits another volume, edition, or set of authors.

CONTENTS

SECTION ONE

Diagnostic Reasoning in the Nursing Domain: Perspective and Process

Doris L. Carnevali

Prologue
A Fable

There once was a land which had been blanketed in a dense fog as long as anyone could remember. Its natives, despite the fog, functioned familiarly and comfortably in their misty country, having been taught the lay of the land by previous generations of residents. When outsiders viewed the territory and the natives functioning there, they found it difficult to recognize what was happening because the shrouding mists made everything so fuzzy and obscure.

The inhabitants of the foggy land traveled daily to an adjoining country whose terrain and language were very much like their own. There, they functioned with and for their neighbors, as had been their tradition and training for many generations. This neighboring land had much less fog, so the landmarks, roads, and activities could be viewed with unhampered clarity. The natives of the clear land, and the tourists who watched the functioning of the immigrant workers, could see more clearly what they did in the foreign land than they could see what they did in their foggy native country. The immigrant workers found the neighbor's land an attractive place to work, with many rewards of status and money, in addition to the sense of tradition and comfort in the activities they were assigned to do.

As time went by, the fog that veiled the homeland of the immigrants finally began to lift. The character of the terrain, the boundaries and the activities of these people in their own domain became increasingly apparent. Tourists who traveled to the once befogged land, and who received services from the natives, began to recognize the different resources and services that

1

were available. More precise maps of the land were developed. Its natural resources were explored and developed. The residents began to find that there was much to keep them occupied within their own land, and there came to be less attraction in traveling to other domains to seek their fortunes. While almost all the residents still commuted to their neighbor's country periodically, when they were needed, many spent more time working at home. New generations were still taught the language, arts and crafts of their neighboring country, but they paid increasing attention to the knowledge of their own language and the skills of their own domain.

A growing pride in their own country emerged. This growing nationalism did not always please the neighbors who wished to continue in the traditional economic and service relationships. Tourists too were initially uncertain about how to travel between the countries and about how to relate differently to the natives in each of the countries. Sometimes, neighboring countries even attempted to discourage tourism into the once foggy land.

Timed passed. Natives, neighbors and tourists became more accustomed to the changes in the country and its people. New traditions and relationships were formed. Trade agreements were established. Commerce between the countries grew, as did tourism and recognition from other domains. The once foggy land of emigrants produced a growing number of artisans, scholars, writers, healers, and persons with associated expertise. The land and its people prospered and grew.

An Analogy

Nursing, like the fabled land, with its shroud of mist, is emerging as a more visible domain among the neighboring health care professions. As nurses themselves are recognizing and developing their discipline, patients and colleagues in other disciplines are coming to acknowledge and use the distinctive perspective and expertise that nurses bring to health care.

Nursing's contribution—its perspective and expertise—is distinguishable in focus and treatment from the delegated medical care, and also from the services that nurses provide for other professions as a part of their traditional role. Certainly, the full extent of the terrain of nursing and its resources have not been explored and mapped; boundaries are still controversial. Nonetheless, the work is progressing steadily. Fewer people now question the existence of a nursing domain—a distinct perspective for nursing diagnosis and treatment.

The changing relationships between nursing and other health disciplines, which resulted from independence in diagnosis and treatment, are not always comforting to any of the participating parties. The uncertainty of many nurses regarding their own domain of knowledge and expertise still presents a foggy, indistinct image to both patients and colleagues, and this image does not encourage appropriate recognition and utilization. Still, growing numbers of nurses are functioning with clarity and confidence in the nursing discipline. Change is taking place slowly—not unusual, considering the numbers of nurses involved, the long traditions so firmly established, and the pressure from others to maintain status quo. Despite this, nursing is emerging in its distinctiveness, as is a critical mass of nurses who are prepared to practice as co-professionals in multi-and interdisciplinary health care systems.

Of Professions and Disciplines

Professions exist in a society because that society recognizes and approves the block of services that a profession gives to the society's members. Accountability for those services and a code of ethics governing the behavior of the members of the profession become a part of the written and unwritten agreement that the profession and the society have with each other in order to ensure the nature of those services.

A *discipline* is accorded a separate identity when other disciplines offer recognition that it:

☐ brings a distinct and characteristic perspective to the viewing of present situations or phenomena

☐ develops a knowledge base to assure growing rigor and expertise needed to validly explain phenomena, and their relationships to that discipline's perspective.

When these two elements are joined into a *Professional Discipline*, the result is a society-approved service based on a discipline-specific perspective and expertise, which is supported by an associated, tested knowledge base.

Nursing has reached a point in its professional evolution where it has a recognized distinct perspective, both in viewing health care situations and in diagnosing and treating health care problems for individuals and groups.

Relationship of Professional Status and Decision Making

The growing importance of skilled diagnostic reasoning in nursing is linked directly to the recognition of the distinct nursing focus in health care. This is not surprising. Health care professionals are hired by clientele (either directly or indirectly, through institutions), for their discipline-based expertise in both diagnosis and treatment. That distinct discipline-specific perspective and expertise are crucial. They come into play the moment the first encounter with client data occurs, when the professional's initial clinical decision is, "What is it important that I as a nurse/physician/dentist/pharmacist . . . notice in this presenting situation?" The decision of noticing or ignoring cues grows out of discipline-based education, training, roles, and experience; and it varies accordingly. Different disciplines train individuals to notice and give significance to varying aspects of a situation, with the same data giving rise to varying directions of thinking for each discipline. The next clinical decision in an encounter is, "How do I classify and explain what it is I am observing as a basis for helping the person to deal with it most effectively?" Again, the explanatory-diagnostic concepts will be discipline-specific.

Because this discipline orientation and knowledge base are so critical to professional practice, the characteristic perspective of nursing—its focus in diagnostic reasoning and treatment decisions—will be the point of departure in this book. After the domain of nursing is described, the components of the process used in making clinical judgements will then be addressed.

CHAPTER ONE

The Nursing Domain for Diagnostic Reasoning

Doris L. Carnevali

OVERVIEW

Nursing's discipline-specific domain for diagnostic reasoning focuses on two major components and their relationships to each other. They are: *Daily Living*, including the environment within which this daily living takes place, and *Functional Health Status*. In *nursing's diagnostic reasoning, these two elements are always viewed in their relationship to each other.*

Within this daily living-health status orientation, nursing's perspective in diagnostic reasoning takes two directions:

the influence that daily living and its environment have on present and future health status

and

the effect that current/potential health status has on daily living and the person's relationship with the environment.

Figure 1–1 illustrates the diagnostic relationships.

DESCRIPTION OF THE ELEMENTS

Daily Living

Nursing's perspective in viewing the daily living of its clientele includes two components: what they do (ADLs) and what they and others (people and things) demand of them in daily living (DDLs).

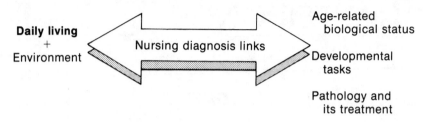

FIG. 1–1. (*Adapted from Carnevali D: Nursing Care Planning, Diagnosis and Management, 3rd ed, Philadelphia, J.B. Lippincott, 1983*)

ADLs, from the nursing view, includes current activities—this minute, this hour, this day, regardless of whether the activities take place in a clinic, operating room, intensive/acute/long term care unit, or in non-institutional settings. This view incorporates previous patterns in the activities of daily living, both preferred and actual, as these are relevent to the presenting situation. But nursing is concerned not only with dimensions of *what is done,* but also with its *significance* to the patient and to other persons who are particularly involved with, or affected by, the activity in question; for example, cooking-eating, income production, sexual activity, and so forth.

Environment

Nursing's concern in diagnostic reasoning and treatment planning tends to focus on the immediate environment in which the person engages in daily living, e.g. the room or units involved in institutional daily living, or the home, neighborhood, school or workplace environments—those aspects of the environment for daily living that are relevant to current or future health status in the presenting problem areas. (A more macro-environmental approach may be undertaken when the health or well-being in ADLs are endangered by the system, but in individual diagnosis and treatment, nursing's focus tends to be more limited).

Functional Health Status

Health status in the nursing domain is viewed as a variable and includes three major components.

Normal Age-Related Biological Status. Nursing is concerned with the normal age-related functioning of all body systems, since they affect the management of daily living as well as patient response to pathology and its treatment.

Developmental Tasks.   Another age-based dimension in the nursing domain is the cluster of developmental tasks associated with the stage of development of the person being diagnosed. Developmental tasks are influenced by the health status of the patient and that of significant others; and, in turn, they affect the approach and response to health-related activities and demands in daily living.

Pathology and Its Treatment.   Pathology is the third dimension of health status in nursing's consideration. Nursing views pathology not only in terms of its alteration of structure and function, but also in terms of the effect these alterations have on developmental tasks, daily living, and the relationship of the person to his environment. Similarly, biomedical diagnosis and treatment are viewed in terms of their effect on the current and potential resources the person can bring to daily living, as well as the alterations in activities and demands generated by the biomedical diagnostic protocols and treatment regimens.

DESCRIPTION OF THE RELATIONSHIPS OF DAILY LIVING AND HEALTH STATUS IN THE NURSING DOMAIN

Daily Living and Its Effects on Health Status

Activities and patterns in daily living affect present and future health status. This is true whether that daily living is taking place at home, work, or school; or in an emergency room, critical care unit, or long-term health-care setting. What may vary is the time lag between the activity in daily living and the resulting health status. Fetal alcohol syndrome has a time lag of weeks or months between the activity of alcohol ingestion by the mother and the observed manifestations in the neonate. Maternal ingestion of DES (diethylstilbesterol) took years to manifest itself in the health status of daughters and possibly sons. Dietary patterns or stress may take months to years to show their effects. On the other hand, in an elderly stroke patient, failure to engage in full extension movements of affected joints can result in contractures within hours or days. Or a more extreme example— failure to maintain a patent airway can cause brain damage in minutes.

On the positive side, good nutrition, exercise and effective management of stress are seen as ways to foster good health status now and in the future. In health care settings, the maintaining of adequate fluids, nutrition, stress management, sensory environments, skin integrity, and airways also contribute to both short-and long-term positive health status. In each instance, an activity of daily living—whether eating, drinking, moving, breathing, or sensing—has affected a person's health in some way.

When daily living and its effect on health status is the focus, nursing's responsibility for making clinical judgments and decisions about treatment is directed to discovering risk factors and signs and symptoms indicating the risk of, or existence of, health problems linked to daily living. Nursing's **data base** will also include an assessment of the person's/family's resources for ongoing effective management of daily living and its environment, as these affect health status. Nursing's **management strategies** will involve helping clients to use their own resources effectively, enhancing underutilized resources where possible, recruiting missing resources, and supplementing or complementing inadequate or missing internal and external resources. It can also involve modification of the activities and demands of daily living as well as the environment to make them more compatible with the existing or projected health status.

In the area of daily living as a way to promote present and future health, the clientele may be presently healthy or ill. There has been a misconception made by some nurses that prevention deals only with healthy persons. It is true that at times this dimension of nursing addresses itself to the needs of essentially healthy people. Here the goal is to gain or safeguard a satisfactory level of health or to achieve better levels, given the internal and external resources available to them. More often, nursing helps those who have existing health problems engage in patterns of daily living that will prevent, delay, or minimize complications and progression of disease as well as promote improved health for the future—again, given the status of internal and external resources available. Further, nursing is as concerned with maintaining wellness in systems unaffected by disease as in those that are. Thus, nursing's attention to living for health is not limited to prevention and maintenance in healthy persons, but extends the same focus to those who are experiencing pathology or trauma.

Nursing's concern with activities and demands of daily living includes not only the individual immediately involved, but also those who are sharing the experience. Most often this is a family group, but it may also include others, such as fellow employees, classmates, residents in shared housing, and others. Their health and effective management of daily living during times of related stress, and their health maintenance is also within nursing's scope of practice. And, where the family is the client, it is the family's immediate support systems that also must be encompassed in nursing's judgments and decision making. In many instances, the individual's or family's health status and well-being are dependent upon the well-being and resources of those around them. There are times when the family is the primary focus of nurses' attention in the maintenance of wellness; parenting, child abuse, juvenile-onset diabetes, and alcoholism are examples. At other times the family is a secondary focus as the nurse attempts to maintain the well-being of its members in order to mobilize them as an external resource to the patient in either acute or long term illness.

Living with Changing Health Status

Throughout a person's life span, structural and functional changes are occurring. Developmental tasks emerge. Some are accomplished and some are not. Normal, age-related, changing health status and developmental tasks are an integral part of nursing's considerations in health care. Variations in structure, function and goals associated with normal developmental stages affect health, risks of disease, activities, and demands of daily living as well as relationships with the environment. In addition, when pathology is present, the person's stage of development and age-related biological status, and the implications these have on health care, must be integrated in nursing's clinical judgments and decision making. Thus, whether helping the clientele plan for maintaining wellness or living with illness, these variables are crucial. Nursing's focus in understanding the client and his patterns of daily living incorporates:

normal age-associated changes in body structure and functioning

developmental tasks in progress

pathology and associated dysfunction as well as the effects of treatment

and

where abnormality and/or dysfunction are present, an integration of the pathology and treatment-related phenomena with the normal age-related factors.

Normal Age-Related Biological Status and Nursing. Daily living patterns and vulnerability to health risks in everyday living change with alternations in body structure and functioning that are normally associated with particular age levels. Some examples will illustrate this.

- ☐ The stage of dentition, the status of teeth, and other parts of the oral cavity go through normal changes from infancy to old age. They affect activities of daily living such as appearance, comfort, nutrition, and communication.
- ☐ Epiphyseal lines in long bones are most fragile during children's growing years, just at a time when rough play activities tend to put them in jeopardy.
- ☐ Teen age boys and girls become capable of reproductive activity well in advance of the maturity required to assume responsibility for effective parenting.
- ☐ Older persons whose balance tends to become more precarious, vision less acute, and gait less agile, also have more fragile bones as cortices thin. They are thus at a much higher risk of falls and fractures in the normal course of activities of daily living.
- ☐ Immune systems have age-associated changes that require consideration in evaluating risks in daily living and responses to illness.

These few examples of age-related changes in structure and functioning illustrate how individuals are at particular risk in terms of their health as they go about their normal lives, and how patterns of daily living are altered to some degree to accomodate the normal age related health status. Few body systems are so stable throughout life that normal age-related changes do not need to be taken into consideration when helping clients, healthy or ill, to plan for effective management of daily living.

Changes in structure and function not only have impact on activities of daily living, but also create different relationships with the environment:

- ☐ Persons with respiratory problems are unusually responsive to air quality.
- ☐ Temperature control is less stable in the very young and the very old. Controls of environmental temperature, types of clothing, hydration, and knowledge of strategies to manage heat gain and loss

become more important. The hypothermic deaths of older people, particularly the poor elderly in cold regions when inflation caused them to cut back on both high priced fuel to warm their external environment and food to stoke their internal furnace, illustrates a changed relationship with the environment and demands that weren't met. The deaths of the old, and occasionally the young, in the 1980 heat wave which occurred in the southwestern United States, offer a similar example of the altered capacity to deal with higher environmental temperatures.

□ Older individuals with normally compromised cardiac function can be essentially immobilized by hilly terrain and/or altitude.

The lack of ability to adjust to one's environment, secondarily to changed structure or function, creates demands for environmental change or some form of added support or protection. The needs for assistance in living with non-supportive environments constitute a domain for nursing judgments and decisions.

Developmental Tasks and Nursing.   Daily living and health are also linked to age-related developmental tasks. According to Erickson, these are:

Stage of Development	Developmental Tasks
Infancy	Trust vs mistrust
Childhood	Autonomy vs doubt
	Iniative vs guilt
	Industry vs inferiority
Adolescence	Identity vs diffusion
Adult	Intimacy vs isolation
	Generativity vs self absorption
	Integrity vs despair
	(Erickson, 1955)

Since these developmental tasks are inseparable from health status and daily living, they too are a part of nursing's concern. An effective achievement of developmental tasks is frequently jeopardized by illness of the individual or of crucial members of the family. The following examples illustrate this:

□ The development of trust can be impaired by hospitalization and treatment where the child feels abandoned by parents. Hospitalization of the mother or caring person can also deter the development of trust.

☐ The developmental task of intimacy can be frustrated by trauma or disease that interferes with sexual capability in young adults, such as the para-and quadriplegics or those suffering from impotence associated with juvenile-onset diabetes. Altered appearance can also deter intimacy.

☐ At mid-life, the adult developmental task is one of productivity. Disabling diseases, such as severe coronary artery disease, can make it difficult if not impossible to achieve the developmental task.

Part of nursing's perspective in making clinical judgements is to take into consideration the developmental tasks associated with the life stages of the patient and the family, and to incorporate these needs as well as others into both the diagnosis and the management plan.*

Pathologic States.   Functional disability secondary to pathology, trauma, or developmental disability tends to create disruptions in usual patterns of daily living. Medical treatment and prescriptions for alterations in lifestyle as well as the location of required care, can compound difficulties in daily living. These dislocations in living occur in some degree whether the person is critically, acutely, or chronically ailing. Nursing's perspective is an important component in health-care management when specifying:

the internal and external resources threatened or lost secondary to the disability and treatment,

the new demands created by the situation,

the arenas of the individual's and family's lifestyle that are threatened or disrupted by these changes,

the resources that can be mobilized to assist in maintaining the most effective and satisfying lifestyle, under the circumstances, for the individual and those important to him.

Each of these areas of specification are affected by the seriousness and intensity of the dysfunction as well as the projected course of events associated with it.

*For more extensive treatment see D. Carnevali, *Nursing Care Planning: Diagnosis and Management* 3rd ed. Philadelphia, J. B. Lippincott, 1983, pp 18–20.

Combining Age-Related Factors and Disability.   A constant consideration in the nursing perspective is the integration of age-related biologic and psychosocial factors into the analysis of the presenting clinical situation. Judgements and decisions are made relative to effective living and health-directed behavior in the presence of disease, disability, and its treatment.

A MODEL FOR NURSING ASSESSMENT, DIAGNOSIS AND MANAGEMENT

A nursing perspective that focuses on patterns of daily living, and the environment in which it takes place, as these are related to health and illness, lends itself to a model that structures;

> areas for data gathering and directions for branching logic
>
> diagnostic categories
>
> prognosis and variables affecting it
>
> management strategy options
>
> criteria for evaluating response to nursing treatment.

Figure 1–2 illustrates one way of visualizing the variables and their relationships.

> Activities Of Daily Living (**ADL**): regularity/frequency of activities and events in daily living and their importance to those involved. Current ADLs (as in institutional care of prescribed changes) and discrepancies from usual/preferred patterns.
>
> Demands Of Daily Living (**DDL**): self expectations plus those held by others that affect activities, choices, or feelings about activities of daily living and demands generated by housing, car, pets, job, environment, and so on.
>
> Internal Resources (**IR**): the status of structure and functional capabilities that can be mobilized to manage ADLs and DDLs. Resources include: strength, endurance, knowledge, skill, desire, courage, and the ability to maintain a satisfying functional sensory environment and the ability to communicate.
>
> External Resources (**ER**): the status of external resources

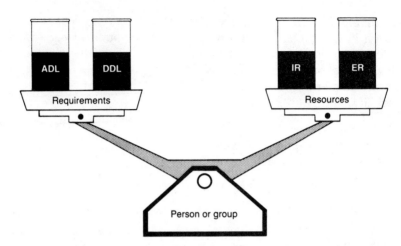

FIG. 1–2.   *A balance model for viewing requirements and resources in daily living and health. (ADL, activities of daily living; DDL, demands of daily living; IR, internal resources; ER, external resources; Adapted from Carnevali D, Patrick M: Nursing Management for the Elderly, Philadelphia, J.B. Lippincott, 1979)*

> that affect health and lifestyle: architecture, people, pets, money, technical/professional services, envirnomental factors, and so forth.

This model proposes that the person, family or group is a fulcrum attempting to maintain a working balance between one arm that contains areas for expenditures of the person's resources, and an opposite one that specifies the nature of the resources available, as these apply to daily living in health and illness. Data for nursing assessment are available in each of these categories. The nature of balance and the aspects that contribute to imbalance constitute the clinical judgment that becomes the nursing diagnosis. The diagnostic statement incorporates both the health status impacting on daily living and the particular area(s) of daily living affected by the particular health problems or issues. (See Chapter 2 p. 49) Variables on either side enable formulation of a prognosis for achieving effective management of daily living for health and participation in health-related behaviors as well as satisfaction with the quality of life that results. (See Chapter 2, p. 49–50) All this then serves as a basis for planning nursing management strategies to deal with activities, demands, internal and external resources in order to bring them into a degree of balance at a level that is or can become tolerable, comfortable, and satisfying to the individual or group involved.

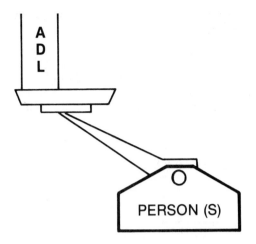

Activities of Daily Living

Patterns of daily activities, usual and preferred, are a crucial element in nursing perspective. This encompasses not only what is done regularly or irregularly, frequently or infrequently, but also the importance of the activity and its timing. Some activities are frequent but unimportant to a person. For example, one person may eat merely to live and may have irregular or unusual eating patterns, while another person lives to eat. Sexual activity may be viewed by the patient/or partner(s) as an important frequent activity; for others it may not. Exercise is seen as vital for some and something to be avoided by others. For a rising professional musician, daily serious practicing is requisite, either enjoyed or looked upon as a duty, but certainly necessary. For the youngster who is being forced to take music lessons, anything that restricts this activity is a delight. Health providers' opinions about what is normal or what "should be" is no substitute for the patient/client's perceptions and observed data.

Data on patterns of daily activity become the basis for clinical decisions as to the aspects of the person's lifestyle, which are:

generators of health directed behaviors or contributors to
predictable loss of health (*e.g.*, occupational noise and
deafness, smoking, and lung cancer),

critical indicators of areas of living that are likely to be
impacted by dysfunction, disease, treatment, or
dislocations associated with treatment (*e.g.*,
institutionalization or travel for treatment),

predictors of ease or difficulties the person will have in

participating in, or complying with, health care management protocols,

descriptors of differences between usual or preferred patterns and demands of daily living, and those required by routines and treatments in health care institutions. (Such differences create uncertainty and need for adjustment and thus new demands for energy)

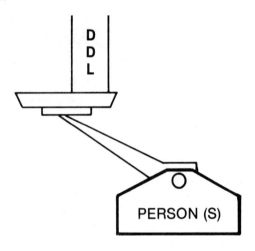

Demands of Daily Living

Demands of daily living represent an element different from activities. This category includes self-expectations as well as the expectations that others can bring to bear upon the person or group that in turn affects lifestyle. These self- and other expectations affect not only what one does, but the style with which it is done, the priorities, the choices, *and* the emotional reactions secondary to those choices. The environment and elements of external resources also generate demands.

Self-Expectations.   Each person or group, at some point in its existence, develops a self-concept and set of self-expectations about a style of living. These self-images (including body image) strongly and pervasively influence choices, priorities, and the style of living under both usual and unusual circumstances. Data about the person in this area can serve to predict the ease or difficulty an individual may have in adjusting to altered status (illness, aging), new diagnostic labels and health care providers' expectations of acceptance of, and compliance with, treatment requirements.

For example, persons who see themselves as athletes may be expected to have difficulty with losses of strength, endurance, or coordination. Those with a self-image of beauty may react more strongly to anything that threatens it—scarring, age, hair loss with chemotherapy. Individuals who have a self-concept of controlling one's self and others can find loss of control, or even threat of this loss, unusually hard to tolerate, while dependent persons find the need to take control equally disconcerting. Some, for whom cognitive prowess is critical to their view of themselves, may find drugs or diseases that alter thinking or communicating a devastating loss.

Data in these areas help to predict and explain the response to presenting health situations and the adjustments that will be required. What will be stressful to one will be no problem to another.

Other Demands of Daily Living.   Human beings have links with people, animals, objects, and activities that generate expectations and obligations: parents, children, siblings, mates, friends, pets, homes, jobs. In turn, these expectations and obligations affect the person's behavior and choices. Additionally, these demands made on the person, whether they are met or unmet, create emotional responses—gratification and pleasure, guilt, anger.

Nursing needs knowledge about specific demands and the composite of the expectations of others, the weight or importance they carry for the person, and the emotional responses generated. It helps in understanding the client's response to health status and health related activities.

Once a client enters a health system, the health care providers also place expectations upon the patient and the family. Some of the expectations that are rather routinely made include:

acceptance of new diagnostic labels and sudden changes in body image,

acceptance of proffered or recommended major treatments,

acceptance, with good grace, of loss of privacy and control over space, information, self, and lifestyle,

compliance with treatment plans and alteration in lifestyle for short or long periods,

engaging in the "good patient" role,

acceptance of unexpected, sometimes unsupportable, financial burdens.

All these and more are health-provider demands that are added regularly to the ongoing demands of daily living.

The nursing perspective requires a valid data base on the specific demands in daily living that the client is experiencing, the extensiveness of the composite demands and the "expense" to the person of meeting them. These data are then viewed in relationship to the data on the presenting health status and management. Such background enables the nurse to make a more accurate interpretation of the patient's response to his presenting health situation. The data also predicts areas of difficulty in participating in health care regimens.

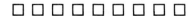

One side of the balance in daily living and health deals with activities and demands in daily living, both routine, ongoing ones and the unusual ones occurring in a current presenting situation. Data collection and clinical judgments about the nature of these elements of the patient/family situation are used in both the diagnostic and management decision areas. They may explain patient/family responses. They document areas in living that are requiring expenditure of resources, which in turn are being influenced by health status. Baseline data on usual or preferred patterns in daily living, when compared to routines in a health care setting and treatment protocols, can be useful in determining discrepancies and may suggest areas where prescribed patient participation or compliance may be difficult or impossible.

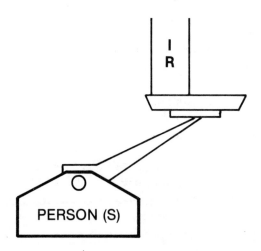

Internal Resources

Internal resources include the status of structure and function that the individual or group has for managing current and predicted activities, and demands in daily living in health-related areas. One way of looking at these resources is in terms of:

Strength: ability and resources to handle physical, mental, emotional work at a given point in time,

Endurance: Stamina, staying power with a work load (physical, intellectual, or emotional),

Sensory Input: Abilities and resources to maintain a functional satisfying sensory environment,

Knowledge: Status of acquired content in the relevant area to be coped with, and level of ability to use that content (*e.g.*, recall, comprehension, application, and so forth.

Desire: Will or motivation to participate

Courage: Risk-taking capacity

Skills: Psychomotor, dexterity, communication, interpersonal.*

Communication: Ability to make one's self understood effectively and acceptably

Internal resources viewed from the perspective of these status areas represent a different approach from that of a body-system organizational framework used in the pathophysiologic approach. The same data on structure and function of body systems still apply, but they are translated into status areas that more particularly address resources for dealing with daily living. Thus, data on structure (*e.g.*, x-ray films or pathology findings) and function (laboratory data, vital signs), become elements in the categories of the internal resources they affect.

The following examples help to illustrate this:

  □ An abnormally low potassium value influences internal resources in several ways. Hypokalemia

* Categories of internal resources. (Adapted from Little D and Carnevali D: Nursing Care Planning, 2nd ed, Philadelphia, J.B. Lippincott, 1976)

results in loss of *strength* and *endurance*. It also can cause change in cardiac function that gives rise to symptoms. These symptoms may create a deficit in *knowledge* regarding the sensations and their meaning, as well as the action to be taken should they occur. Potassium replacement therapy may give rise to other deficits in *knowledge* on how to take the drug as well as a possible deficit in *desire* to take a medication on an ongoing basis that tastes bad and may cause gastric distress.

☐ Among those of advanced age, changes in vision, hearing, taste, and smell predict decreased internal resources for maintaining an adequate sensory environment for safe and effective living.

☐ At the other end of the age continuum is the failure-to-thrive syndrome secondary to the lack of internal resources of the infant to mobilize sufficient, appropriate sensory stimulation of touch, sight, and sound for a satisfactory *sensory environment*.

Diagnostic tests and treatment protocols prescribed by other disciplines and their outcomes also need to be viewed in terms of their influences on internal resources for both short or long periods of time. Some treatments will immediately improve internal resources (*e.g.*, oxygen, fluids, relief of obstructed airway), while others will predictably decrease them either temporarily or on a long-term basis (*e.g.*, surgery, radiation, chemotherapy, side effects of medications).

The nursing viewpoint requires an accurate data base on the status of internal resources and the variables that are affecting them. These findings too are then examined from the perspective of the presenting health situation with the purpose of determining the individual's or group's internal resources for meeting the activities and demands of daily living.

In nursing, it is important to examine not only deficits in internal resources, but strengths as well. In many instances, strengths are available that may not have been recognized, or may be underutilized. This is an indicator that it is possible or desirable to increase demands and activities of daily living in order to more fully use the available resources.

External Resources

External resources are factors, forces, conditions, and systems outside the individual or group that influence their health or health-

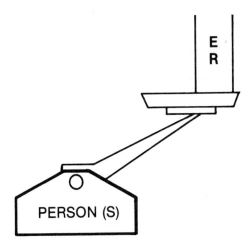

related patterns of daily living. Some categories of external resources are:

> architecture, air and water quality, employment, governmental and other bureaucratic agencies, housing, industry, money, neighborhood, people, pets, services, supplies, technology, terrain, transportation . . .

This list obviously could be very long.

The nursing perspective requires an awareness of several variables in order to understand the relationship between external resources and the person or group. Past, present and future orientations are needed, given the dynamic nature of health and daily living. Another important caveat is the difference between the perceptions of the client and those of the nurse in value-related judgments about external resources. Questions that help a nurse gain perception of the external factors are as follows:

- ☐ What external factors are seen as influencing the presenting health situation? (Consider home, community and institutional settings, as these are potentially involved).
- ☐ Which factors are seen as supportive? As nonsupportive?
- ☐ What resources is the patient using? Effectively? With satisfaction?
- ☐ What else is seen as being needed? Is it available? Will

different resources be needed later, given the prognosis?

☐ What barriers need to be eliminated or overcome? What can't be overcome? How does this affect the prognosis? The treatment plan?

☐ What resources are acceptable to the clientele? Which ones are unacceptable? (The latter is important because resources seen by the client as unacceptable may become nonsupportive forces, rather than the supportive forces they were intended to be).

Given the high costs of health care, the contraints on staffing, and the professional's time with patients, the reality of the situation finds nurses, more often than not, being forced to deal with needs of patients deemed to have the highest priority, while ignoring or delaying attention to less urgent problems or issues. Where high priority care is a necessity, it tends to dictate the focus in viewing external resources. The following are examples.

☐ Where *strength* and *endurance* are impaired, external resources affecting mobility in managing activities and demands of daily living become a priority focus—stairs, terrain, distance to the bathroom or kitchen, nearness of stores, transportation, physical assistance, and so forth,

☐ Nurses in critical care units of teaching hospitals often find that the learning needs and research interests of the many categories of medical personnel who should constitute a professional service resource to the patient generate, instead, excessive demands in daily living for individuals whose endurance is minimal. These professional resources then have become a demanding external force that nurses monitor and control for the critically ill patient's well-being.

It is important for nurses to maintain an awareness that *external resources* are a primary source of demands of daily living. A home or apartment is a resource; it also generates demands. Health care providers are important external resources; they too create demands of their own on the patient and the family. A dog can offer companionship and incentive to go walking and move about; he also presents demands. Family, often a major form of support in illness, is also a prime locus for demands. Employment settings, schools, and the groups in the person's network are other resources, but each places demands on the patient that affects his response. These are important factors the nursing perspective takes into consideration when making clinical judgments about the relationship of health and daily living.

SUMMARY

This book was conceived on the premise that nursing is a professional discipline, that it brings a valued service to society, and that this service grows out of a distinct, recognizable perspective in viewing health and health care. It is this distinct focus that determines the areas of responsibility for clinical judgments and decisions in the nursing domain, as contrasted with those that the nurses will make in the biomedical domain as a part of the delegated functions they incorporate in their role.

Nursing's orientation to diagnostic reasoning and treatment decisions in health care is concerned with the patterns of daily living and its environment, as these affect health and are affected by changes in health status. Diagnostic statements will integrate clinical judgments about the relationships between activities and demands, on the one hand, and the internal and external resources to meet these expenditures, on the other. The diagnostic reasoning process used to arrive at valid clinical judgments and plan for effective health care management is a generic one shared by all health care disciplines engaged in these tasks. What varies is the distinct perspective nursing brings, the data it needs to arrive at these judgments and decisions, the categories of problem classification, the strategies for treatment, and the variables used to evaluate patient response.

BIBLIOGRAPHY

Bruhn J and Cordova FD: A developmental approach to learning wellness behavior: Infancy to adolescence. Health Values 6:246–254, 1977

Carnevali D: Nursing Care Planning: Diagnosis and Management, 3rd ed. Philadelphia, JB Lippincott, 1983

Carnevali D, Patrick M: Nursing Management for the Elderly, Philadelphia, JB Lippincott, 1979

Dickelmann N: Emotional tasks of the middle adult. Am J Nurs 75:997–1001, 1975

Dickelmann N: Primary Health Care of the Well Adult. New York, McGraw-Hill, 1977

Erickson EH: Growth and crises of the "healthy personality." In Kluckhon C, Murray HA, Scheider DM (eds): Personality in Nature, Society and Culture, pp 185–225. New York, Alfred A Knopf, 1955

Erickson EH: Childhood and society, in Eight Stages of Man, 2nd ed. New York, WW Norton, 1963

Goldman R: Aging changes in structure and function. In Carnevali D, Patrick M: Nursing Management for the Elderly. Philadelphia, JB Lippincott, 1979

Kim MJ and Moritz DA: Nursing diagnosis and nursing theory. In Classification of Nursing Diagnosis, pp 214–272. New York, McGraw-Hill, 1982

LaVeck PJ: Developmental reactions in young adulthood. In Kalman M, Davis A (eds): New Dimensions in Mental Health—Psychiatric Nursing, rev ed, pp 129–154. New York, McGraw-Hill, 1974

Little D and Carnevali D: Nursing Care Planning, 2nd ed. Philadelphia, JB Lippincott, 1976

Moore JA: Developmental reactions in middle years. In Kalkman M, Davis A (eds): New Dimensions in Mental Health—Psychiatric Nursing, rev ed. New York, McGraw-Hill, 1974

Orem DE: Nursing: Concepts of Practice. New York, McGraw-Hill, 1971

Patrick M: The elderly and their responses to aging, pp 41–52. In Carnevali D, Patrick M: Nursing Management for the Elderly. Philadelphia, JB Lippincott, 1979

Stevens B: Nursing Theory, Analysis, Application, Evaluation. Boston, Little, Brown & Co, 1979

Tolsdorf CC: Social networks, support, and coping. Fam Process 15:407–418, 1976

Yarrow MR: Appraising environments. In Williams RH (ed): The Process of Aging, vol 1, pp 201–222. New York, Atherton Press, 1963

CHAPTER TWO

THE DIAGNOSTIC REASONING PROCESS

Doris L. Carnevali

Skillful use of the diagnostic reasoning process in identifying health-related problems is the foundation of professional health care. The technical competence needed to carry out the decisions effectively is important, of course, but unless this is preceded by accurate clinical judgments and decisions, it can be useless if not outright dangerous. Consumers of health care do not seek the services of professionals just for the actions they take, but for the professional judgments on which those actions are based. This is as true in nursing as in all other professional fields–medicine, law, education, pharmacy, social work, dentistry. Cost-effective safe nursing requires accurate clinical judgments and, as a basis for treatment, decisions in the nursing domain, as surely as in any other health care discipline.

NURSES COMMONLY DIAGNOSE IN TWO DOMAINS

Tradition and patient well-being require the nurse to be competent enough to engage in diagnostic reasoning and to make treatment decisions in at least two disciplines—nursing and medicine. In the nursing field, nurses have *primary accountability* for making judgments regarding the status of the patient and his family's daily living as it affects or is affected by their health. And once these judgments have been made, they develop treatment plans aimed at helping the individual and family manage effectively the health-related activities and demands of daily living, given their presenting circumstances.

In the biomedical domain, on the other hand, nurses have *delegated responsibility* to make accurate, appropriate clinical judgments on

25

the patients' pathophysiologic/health status. From these judgments regarding the patients' health status, nurses decide whether to

> recommend that the patient continue in self care,*
>
> retain under nursing management,*
>
> refer to physician for medical diagnosis and treatment,*
>
> retain under existing medical regimen, or seek consultation from physician on altering medical treatment regimen

Whatever the domain for professional practice, the diagnostic reasoning process used to arrive at clinical judgments regarding patient status is the same. It is used comparably in each of the health care disciplines. There is economy for nurses in considering the diagnostic reasoning and treatment decision-making processes as generic. One need not change the components or sequence of steps in critical-thinking and data gathering; one need only change the discipline-specific perspective.

OVERVIEW OF THE DIAGNOSTIC REASONING PROCESS

The diagnostic reasoning process is a complex observation-critical, thinking-data gathering process used to identify and classify phenomena that are encountered in presenting clinical situations. This classification with associated labelling is not an end in itself, but a means to an end. It provides the foundation of recognition and knowledge of the nature of the phenomena being observed. This classification and the knowledge associated with it, in turn shape the decisions on treatment regimens that can be undertaken to produce a desired outcome in patient/family response. So, the end point of diagnosis is professional treatment that is rationally predicted to contribute to patient's or family's well-being in specific problem areas.

The diagnostic reasoning process is an indivisible mixture of non-patient-related factors that shape the diagnostician's observation and thinking, the elements of the process, and the sequence. In and of itself, the diagnostic reasoning process is complex, but its complexity is compounded by the reality that the diagnostician is rarely apply-

* Decisions made by nurses working in private practice, schools, industry, clinics in senior centers, long term care with minimal M.D. presence, home care, HMO/ambulatory care clinics with RN, phone health care services, and so forth.

ing the process to just one presenting problem. Each clinical situation encountered for diagnostic purposes presents the liklihood that multiple problems co-exist and are manifesting themselves in some way in the data search field. Thus the process, as it is actually used, more often than not, involves dealing with multiple co-existing problem areas. It is therefore much less linear and simplistic than step-type diagrams would suggest. Still, to understand it as a basis for improving one's diagnostic expertise, one must begin with the basics, even as one accepts that this is an oversimplification of the complexity of its realistic application.

It is on the basis of this premise that the discussion of the diagnostic reasoning process is undertaken in terms of its basic elements, influencing features, and logical sequencing. The overview will first briefly identify each of these areas with more complete treatment of each of them following later in the chapter.

Factors Affecting Diagnostic Reasoning

There are some factors outside the actual clinician-patient encounter that have the potential for profoundly affecting the diagnostic reasoning that is carried out. An awareness of them may help the diagnostician put them into perspective, use them effectively, and perhaps neutralize some of the potentially biasing forces. The factors that have been identified as modifying diagnostic reasoning fall into three major categories:

□ the nature and background of the diagnostician
□ the nature of the setting
□ the nature of the diagnostic task

These factors cannot be viewed as elements in the diagnostic reasoning process, yet their influence is so powerful that no understanding of diagnostic reasoning can be undertaken without considering them.

Elements of the Diagnostic Reasoning Process

The diagnostic reasoning process is itself made up of a series of elements. One might call them a pattern of steps, and on paper the logic of this sequence seems obvious. In actual practice, the blurring of steps and the modifications of sequence may make the process seem less clear cut as the diagnostician deals with myriads of data, high levels of ambiguity, and multiple potential problem areas concurrently. Thus, our choice is to describe elements and a potential pattern of use rather than rigid steps in the process.

The elements and the "logical" order of occurrence are shown in Figure 2–1. Each of these elements is discussed in some detail later in the chapter.

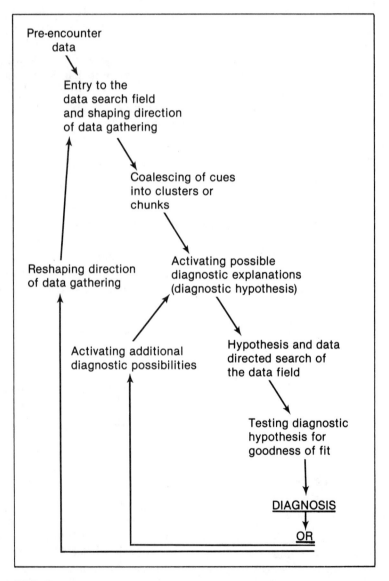

FIG. 2–1.

Level of Awareness as a
Feature of Diagnostic Reasoning

The textbook picture of diagnostic reasoning is that of a consciously logical collection of data, consideration of alternative explanations, and an ultimate choice of classification for what is observed. Clinical practice is again at odds with the textbook picture. Experienced clinicians make many judgments without having a conscious knowledge of which cues were used, how they were clustered, and what weight were given to them. The recognition of a problem or the certainty that a problem does not exist seems at times to pop into one's awareness. On occasion, retrospective analysis allows one to restructure the process and cues used, but not always. This intuitive approach happens with enough frequency that it cannot be ignored.

Berne described four methods for arriving at judgments, only one of which was the conscious, logical derivation of diagnoses from data. The three others involved:

> judgments based on preconscious, preverbal, sensory observations which *could* be translated retrospectively into words and recorded
>
> a subconscious process which may *never* be made conscious, but is presumably based on preconscious sensory input, and
>
> an unknown process by which the diagnostician comes to the judgment without being able to explain to himself or others how he knows it to be true.
>
> (Berne, 1977)

Others too have stressed the need for untrammelled creativity and intuition, particularly in the early stages of problem identification when information about the presenting situation is, of necessity, indefinite and incomplete. (Popper, 1959; Style, 1979, p. 73)

While acknowledging this preconscious, unconscious pattern of hypothesis activation, other researchers take the view that the mystery of human thinking in problem recognition may be more illusory than real. They suggest that the portions that can't be verbalized model closely those that can. (Kassirer and Gorry, 1978, p. 255). Knowledge, previous experience, subtle low-amplitude cues, and inadequacy of language to describe input must all play a part in the appearance of diagnoses that are not consciously activated.

Summary

Diagnostic reasoning then is a complex, sometimes unconscious, integration of critical-thinking, and data-collecting processes that clinicians use to identify and classify phenomena in presenting clinical situations. It is the necessary foundation for subsequent treatment decisions. To understand and gain expertise in diagnostic skills, it is helpful to consider the diagnostic reasoning process in terms of its elements, sequence and influencing factors. At the same time, it is important to acknowledge that in its clinical application—though all these elements are present—the process becomes a much more complex one.

One eminent Swedish physician, Biörck, described the clinician's art as one of making a tremendous number of clinical judgments each day based on indequate, often ambiguous data, and under pressure of time and of carrying out this task with the outward appearance of calmness, dedication and interpersonal warmth. (Biörck 1977, p. 146) No small task!

THE DIAGNOSTICIAN, THE TASK, AND THE SETTING AS INFLUENCES ON DIAGNOSTIC REASONING

Rather obviously, the actual use of the diagnostic reasoning process is influenced by the expertise of the individual diagnostician. It is also profoundly affected by diagnostician characteristics. Other than diagnostic skills per se, the nature of the diagnostic task and the setting in which diagnosis take place also affect the diagnostic process.

The Diagnostician

Just as a patient is an individual with traits similar to most people but with a unique composite of background and responses, so also are diagnosticians. They hold much in common with all other diagnosticians, but there are distinctive influencing characteristics as well. It is wise for the diagnostician to have this self-awareness and to be conscious of the way in which background and other personal factors shape diagnostic reasoning style.

Discipline. The clinician's specific discipline is a major force in shaping diagnostic perspective and style. Each clinical discipline, and often subspecialty, trains its members to view a presenting clinical situation from that discipline-specific or speciality-specific perspective. Each discipline trains its practitioners to use differing data collection strategies and diagnostic protocols. Thus a physician, dentist, nurse, pharmacist and social worker, all viewing the same patient, will approach diagnosis on the basis of their own discipline-specific training.

An example of differences in physician–nurse approaches to a presenting situation may serve to illustrate. The physician, on learning that a patient is experiencing ongoing "depression," gathers data to determine whether the antecedent events and current signs and symptoms represent reactive/exogenous depression for which antidepressants are contraindicated, or endogenous depression requiring medication for its management. Nurses, with a daily living orientation, would have a complementary perspective. They would look to history and immediate antecedent events, the current activities and demands of daily living being altered by change in internal resources involving emotional-physical strength and endurance as well as changes in relationships with external resources—persons, things, use of systems. This too is a basis for treatment decisions in the kind of nursing treatment that would be appropriate and therapeutic.

It is wise in both multidisciplinary and interdisciplinary practice, for clinicians in differing disciplines to be aware of both the limitations and richness of diagnostic perspective and skills that are derived from the varying discipline-specific training and experience of others. Such training and focused experience generates both blinders and extraordinary vision in terms of noticing cues and organizing and interpreting them.

In this area of discipline-specific orientation to diagnostic reasoning, nurses suffer from an identity crisis other disciplines do not experience. Other disciplines tend to see nursing's diagnostic orientation as extensions (at a more elementary or basic level) of their own. And currently, more practicing nurses have been trained to diagnose within the pathophysiologic, psycho-pathologic models as opposed to a daily living model. The extent to which the pathological model has dominated nursing cue perception is illustrated by Gordon's deliberate use of postoperative complications rather than nursing diagnostic categories to test diagnostic strategy in nurses. She felt nurses would be more familiar with and able to articulate their strategy with a pathologically-based situation. (Gordon, 1980) It is a fact of life that nurses must diagnose regularly in both the biomedical and nursing domains as a part of their professional role. This places a double burden to become safely competent as a physician adjunct when diagnosing in the biomedical domain and to be expert and visible when diagnosing within the nursing domain.

One's discipline-specific training and experience then, tends to pre-set the cues one will notice, the vocabulary that will be used to describe cues, the diagnostic concepts that will be used to organize, classify and explain the data as well as the diagnostic labels that will be assigned. This is a strong and pervasive influence on diagnostic behavior.

Experience Level of the Diagnostician. There are certain patterns of characteristics in diagnostic behavior associated with the amount of time the clinician has been practicing and the stage of development in diagnostic expertise the clinician has achieved. These patterns of differences tend not to be discipline-specific. Tanner describes the nature of these variables in diagnostic behavior associated with the stage of diagnostic development in Section 2 of this book. It can be seen that the stage of development in diagnostic expertise of any given clinician will have a marked effect on the data-gathering behavior, the diagnostic reasoning patterns and the diagnoses that are produced.

Personal Variability. In addition to discipline and experience/expertise factors, there are also individual variables that influence the diagnostic process. One of these variables has to do with the diagnostician's storage of knowledge and experience in long-term memory. The other relates to the diagnostician's mental and physical status at the time diagnostic reasoning is undertaken.

Memory. What is stored in memory and how it is stored, is a personal variable. Recency, intensity, and frequency of patient events will influence both what one is prepared to notice and how one interprets it. This is particularly true for the person how has stored these experiences only in *episodic long term memory.* (see pp. 45–70). Further, the number of diagnostic concepts, their quality and sharpness, and the organizational system used in storing this knowledge in semantic long-term memory for diagnostic retrieval, will actually determine what the clinician is able to diagnose. One cannot diagnose what one does not recognize or understand. The amount and precision of cross referencing or cross linkage between related concepts will determine the degree of expertise the clinician is able to achieve. It is true that some of the discipline content committed to long-term memory and the discipline-specific system for storage can be assured through exposure to education and training—it can be tested through licensing examinations. Still, the analytic, organizational, and language skills, as well as the energy individual clinicians devote to this aspect of their professional competency, are very personal qualities. Hence there are individual differences in diagnostic capabilities despite comparability of training. Within the individual clinician, the level of diagnostic competence varies with the diagnostic task. Tasks that fall outside the diagnostician's common areas of experience and expertise will result in a drop in diagnostic efficiency. An unfamiliar diagnostic task is not matched by the content in long-term memory or by the skill of retrieval, both of which are available in the clinician's more practiced areas. Thus, diagnostic ability in *any* diagnostician is a profile of levels, not a steady state.

The diagnostician's *physical, mental and emotional state* at the time the diagnostic reasoning is undertaken is another individual variable. High levels of anxiety and/or fatigue can both narrow the data-search field and encourage premature closure in making a diagnosis. Feeling an urgent need to make a speedy diagnosis—either because of urgent patient status, expectations by self or others, or pressure of additional tasks, will also affect the nature of search of the data field and the diagnostic reasoning process.

In summary, individual differences is use of diagnostic reasoning will be influenced by the way in which knowledge and experience are stored in long-term memory for diagnostic purposes. It will also be influenced by the goodness of fit between the area of diagnostic expertise and experience of the diagnostician and the diagnostic tasks being presented by the patient. Even within an individual diagnostician, diagnostic efficiency and skill may vary widely. Finally data gathering and diagnostic reasoning are shaped by the physical, mental, and emotional status of the diagnostician at the time of encountering the diagnostic task.

The Setting

The setting within which the diagnosing takes place exerts its own influence over diagnostic behavior. Some of the factors that shape diagnosticians' activities are: structural characteristics, equipment, role expectations, and predominate clientele.

Physical structure and *equipment* directly shape the kind of data that is available and probably influence indirectly the kind of data and diagnoses that are valued. Nurses working as patient phone consultants in HMO's, and other types of ambulatory-care settings have their data field shaped by the fact that their mechanical data-gathering device is the telephone and their only communication route for structuring and receiving patient data is *auditory.* Thus, they tune in to auditory cues and engage in strategies to help patients translate non-auditory cues into words or sounds. The patient is physically located at some distance so the data search field may give greater emphasis to cues of potential for self-assessment and resources for self-care, including transportation to the health care setting, if needed. In Section 3, McCorkle describes another approach to initial data gathering and diagnosis by phone, where the setting is noninstitutional. Mitchell, in her chapter on diagnostic reasoning in a critical care setting, cites the influence of sophisticated technology. Here the diagnosticians' data field includes, not only a presenting patient who can be seen, heard and touched externally, but whose internal states are being monitored in a refined fashion—with numerical or graphic data that can even be captured on paper to prevent loss and to show trends or patterns. Other clinical settings build in differing mechanical means of data collection with the expectation that they will be used by diagnosticians functioning in these areas. The result is that different data bases emerge and, eventually, different data come to be valued by diagnosticians who work there on an ongoing basis. Thus, these forces in the setting shape diagnostic behavior.

Another setting-based force is *role expectations.* In some ambulatory care settings, quotas are set as to the number of patients to be seen per time period. In in-house settings, case loads serve this same function. Expectations as to who has the legitimate right to function overtly as a diagnostician, and the time and control of practice allowed for diagnostic activities, are other setting-based forces shaping diagnostic behavior. In the nursing field the "appears to be" preface to a diagnosis made by a nurse testifies to the level of legitimacy for diagnosis made by nurses. A look at job descriptions, assignments that allocate time for physical tasks, and delegated medical treatments but that allocate none for nursing's assessment and diagnosis is another example of the role expectations that nursing systems have for their own clinicians. Such setting-based role expectations cannot help but shape nurses' diagnostic behavior.

A third major setting-based influence is the type of *clientele that predominate* numerically in a setting. The prevailing clientele and associated types of health issues or problems tend to mold the observing and thinking behavior of clinicians who practice in this setting. Over time they will come to pay attention to certain types of cues while ignoring others; they will entertain certain diagnoses and not others. The prevailing clientele can also skew the way diagnosticians interpret cues. One hears, not too infrequently, of diabetics who are unfortunate enough to go out of control in a public place being placed in the "drunk tank" of the municipal jail. That wouldn't happen in a diabetic clinic where the clinicians see more unstable diabetics than they do severe chronic alcoholics. Similarly, somatic diseases may tend to be recognized less quickly in a psychiatric unit while the reverse may be true in an acute-care setting of a general hospital.

Further, the greater the discrepancy between the characteristics of the diagnostician and the patient, the greater the use of stereotypes and associated risks for inaccurate interpretation of data. Where the prevailing clientele is markedly different from the diagnosticians in economic status, ethnic and cultural background, language, lifestyle, these differences can shape diagnostic behavior. (Scheff, 1965, pp. 143–144)

Thus the equipment and physical structure of the setting, the systems, role expectations, and the prevailing clientele of the setting all tend to shape diagnostic reasoning somewhat independently of the actual data and problem being presented by the patient.

The Diagnostic Task

The diagnostic task itself is to infer and classify the status of the patient on the basis of whatever data are present and available to the diagnostician.

Under most circumstances the diagnostician is required to enter into an encounter with a presenting patient situation—a disconcertingly open data field with a constellation of cues never before totally experienced in all its dimensions. It is replete with uncertainty as to whether the most urgent and important problems to be diagnosed will present themselves with sufficient cues or cues of sufficient amplitude and clarity to be noticed and recognized. There will be cues that could be indicators of more than one diagnosis. There will also be the ambiguity of missing (or at least unrecognized) cues needed to reach a particular diagnosis. Cues that are relevant to problems requiring recognition and treatment are mingled with even greater numbers of "irrelevant" cues.

The diagnostician's challenge then is to find a known starting point and to move into, and make order out of, this uncertain ambiguous world of cues—to collect, sort out, and organize them, to gradually delimit the search spaces, to find the normals, and gradually move to the terminal point of assigning diagnostic classification and deciding on treatment options.

At times there are enough "related" clear cues to permit the diagnostician to be comfortable in assigning a "definite"diagnostic label to them. More often, there are not enough cues or cues of the "required" kind to offer this comfortable diagnostic certainty, and the diagnostician is required to live with the irreducible uncertainty of too general a diagnosis, too provisional a diagnosis, or no diagnosis at all.

There is no question that this complex, probabalistic, uncertain task of moving from wide open beginnings and the responsibility of producing valid diagnoses within the time constraints (repeated many times each day) generates high cognitive strains on the diagnostician. (Elstein et al, 1978, p. 65) The attempts to reduce this cognitive strain are a major force influencing the styles and strategies used in the diagnostic reasoning process.

Summary

In the preceding pages, we have examined an overview of the structure of diagnostic reasoning as well as some of the major factors, external and internal (to the diagnostician), that tend to shape the way in which the elements will actually be implemented clinically. It was hoped that by examining these forces first the reader would become aware that diagnostic reasoning behavior is anything but a cut-and-dried stereotyped activity, identical in all diagnosticians and altered only by the patient's presenting situation.

Perhaps by alerting the student, clinician-diagnostician, the teacher of future diagnosticians, and the supervisors of practicing diagnosticians, to the variables affecting diagnostic behavior, the process can be approached with greater realism and honesty. Conditions that contribute to the biasing or skewing of diagnostic behavior can be acknowledged and activities to neutralize biasing features can be undertaken where this is possible. Where nothing can be changed, at least the influences and potential outcomes can be identified and recognized for what they are and what they do.

ELEMENTS OF THE DIAGNOSTIC REASONING PROCESS

The nature of the elements in and of themselves need to be understood before they are viewed either as a sequence or a whole. Only then can they be utilized most effectively.

Pre-encounter Patient Data

One of the ways in which diagnosticians reduce cognitive strain is to set early limits on the data space by using patient data available before the actual one-to-one encounter with the patient occurs. Sex and age are units of data frequently used in biomedical diagnosis to narrow the field. (Kassirer and Gorry, 1978, p. 247) This is logical; there is pathophysiology that is limited to males or to females, or more likely to occur in one sex than in the other. Similarly, some conditions are impossible or unlikely in certain ages while others are a high risk at certain ages. Each of these considerations takes some possibilities out of consideration and decreases or increases the probabilities of others, thus giving some beginning reduction of the total open-endedness of the presenting situation.

In Section 3 of the book the reader should contrast the data that the clinicians would prefer to have, or actually use, to begin to raise some probabilities of daily living problems or to reduce the probability of others. For example, Simmons values pre-encounter data on age and sex to help her predict increased or reduced risk of nutritional problems for persons with end-stage renal disease. McCorkle, in dealing with persons in the end stages of oncologic disease, does not see age and sex as altering probabilities of problems in daily living with metastatic disease, but does want data on tumor-type, biomedical treatment regimen, the time interval since the patient knew of the diagnosis, the name of the treating physician, and the source of referral. Any or all of these are useful to her in shaping her data search and setting initial probabilities for diagnosis. Mitchell, in a critical care setting, gives priority to data indicating status of biologic stability.

It is wise for diagnosticians to be aware of pre-encounter data that they tend to have available or to seek out, and how they use these data to alter their data gathering and to shape consideration of diagnostic possibilities.

Types of Cues in the Presenting Situation

The presenting situation contains cues of several levels of interest and varying uses to the clinician. These can include cues indicating: 1) *risks* of health problems, 2) strength, resources and health or "normality", 3) the presence of problems and 4) many that are seen to be irrelevant, at least from the given clinician's discipline perspective.

Risk Indicators. Cues associated with risk factors signal that a problem is more likely to occur than if these were not present. They also suggest that, should the problem occur, it will be complicated by their presence and therefore, will be more difficult to manage. For example, prospective parents who were abused as children, very young women who are single parents, and those with uncertain financial resources are more likely to be child abusers in their parenting. The presence of cues in more than one of these variables would increase the risk that child abuse will be a problem for the parent and the child. In another example, postoperative patients who are older, obese, smoking, and who have had a general anesthesia and an incision on or close to the chest, are at a higher risk for respiratory complications postoperatively than those who do not present with these indicators. Persons who have adopted a low-income transient lifestyle—the "Kings of the Road"—tend to have precarious housing and eating resources at all times, and are particularly vulnerable in the cold seasons and in recessions.

Cues identifying risk factors may be present in the persons themselves, in their activities of daily living, in the demands of daily living in their environment, and in the status of their external resources. (See Chapter 1, pp. 20–22) Data indicating the presence or absence of risk factors will tend to shape subsequent search areas.

Indicators of Strength.   Another type of cue that is available in the presenting search space is that indicating a high level of strength and available useable resources. From any discipline perspective, it is as important to determine health and effectiveness in living as it is to discover disease and deficits in functional capacity or resources. Many cues are indicators of normality, strength, and adequacy of resources. These become useful in ruling out problems, in predicting prognosis, and in selecting treatment options.

Signs and Symptoms.   While risk factors suggest the possibility or probability of the existence of problems, signs and symptoms are indicators of their actual presence. The terms signs and symptoms have been so closely associated with pathology that some nurses are reluctant to use them in the more generic sense of being *objective and subjective manifestations of any existing health problem*. This is the meaning these terms will have throughout the book.

Symptoms are subjectively reported data. They are indicators of the person's perception of health experiences they have had or are having. "Subjective data" is a synonym for symptom. Symptoms or subjective data may come from the primary source (the patient), and most often do. However, they may also come from secondary sources—people who have been or are sharing the health problem or situation with the patient. Such persons may also give primary subjective data based on their perceptions of what the situation is and what they themselves are experiencing.

Signs are the observable cues that indicate the existence of a problem. "Objective data" is a synonym for signs. Cues that are categorized as objective data can be received through any sense organ directly from the person(s) in the search field. They may also be received indirectly through data via monitors or reports of patient functioning. Signs are used to: 1) confirm reported symptoms and 2) to lend direction to a search for associated subjective data.

Irrelevant Cues.   In any clinical encounter many cues that are not seen as being relevant to understanding the person's health situation will be present. Relevance and significance of cues are in the eye of the beholder. This is true whether the beholder is the patient, those around him, or the clinician. For the clinician, relevance will tend to be discipline-specific. For example, the kind of shoes a person is wearing would tend to be more significant to a podiatrist, a pediatrician, an orthopedist, a geriatrician, at times a nurse, and perhaps a social worker. Shoes probably would not seem significant to a dentist or a pharmacist.

The art in making accurate clinical judgments has its foundation in this early stage of noticing and lending significance to appropriate cues. And, given the discipline-related biases when viewing cues for relevance, there is, in most settings, a sound rationale for interdisciplinary practice.

Entry to the Data Field

The initial direct encounter with the patient and the presenting data search field requires that the diagnostician opt for a known starting point. This may be discipline-or speciality-specific, such as the dentist's initial question about any problems with one's teeth, or the pharmacist starting with currently prescribed drugs. It could also be determined by the nature and urgency of problems the patient presents with, such as airway obstruction, burns, onset of labor, cardiac arrest, seriously contemplated suicide, or rape.

Under usual circumstances, given the clientele the diagnosticians see, they usually have a repertoire of initial strategies for entering the data search field—a quick top-to-toe scanning or observation of particular areas of the patient accompanied by a verbal statement or question that structures the verbal cues the client begins with. Often the "chief complaint" is the point of departure with ambulatory care clientele on an initial visit. For those who haven been previously seen and assessed, the initial focus may be on what has changed since the previous contact. Clinicians writing in the third section of this book use differing strategies for entering the data field, appropriate to their clientele's health status and problem areas.

Not to be overlooked is the kind of disrobing or body exposure of the patient. This too structures the kind of data available as well as expectations the patient has about data the diagnostician wants. For example, Blainey, in Section 3, always want shoes and stockings removed when she sees her diabetic clients. They know she sees feet as important and this fact structures cues they are prepared to provide.

The entry to the data field involves an immediate scanning to determine what urgent priorities may be present. This is followed by strategies to guide the patient to present data that begin to lend direction to subsequent shaping of problem areas and ruling out of problems in which stressors are absent or resources are sufficient for the patient to manage without professional intervention.

Beyond the entry to the data field and the opening structure of the data collection, the early data collection can follow a generalized "standard" pattern that is the norm of one's discipline, or it can take on an early focus toward known high-risk areas. In either case the data that are taken in tend to coalesce into clusters in short-term memory. In turn, single cues or clusters lead to the next stage in the diagnostic reasoning process—that of considering diagnostic possibilities and setting further boundaries around problem areas.

Hypothesis Activation

The use of the term "hypothesis activation" for this early step in problem identification might be viewed as creating unnecessary jargon. Actually it is a precise term used with a definite purpose. The word "hypothesis" is used to maintain the caution that *early labels are and must be tentative*, open to change. When there is so much pressure to see the next patient, to get the work done, the temptation to decide quickly and gain closure is strong. And of course there are times when diagnoses must be established quickly or patients will suffer. On the other hand, treating early diagnoses as hypotheses, as tentative problems labels that are open to change, can help to avoid missed diagnoses and misdiagnosis. The word "activation" accurately describes the initiative and cerebral activity in retrieving the stored knowledge that is essential for effective diagnosis.

All this suggests that the first step in moving toward an organization of random cues in a presenting situation to form a useable data base is not merely a routinized data-collection and recording activity. In early stages of teaching the assessment-diagnostic process, schools for health professionals establish routine data-collection patterns in order to develop systematic approaches in their novice clinicians. Novices are also taught to hold judgment in abeyance until the bulk of the data are in. Some students and clinicians remain at this level of development. It is not, however, the typical approach used by experienced clinicians in actual practice. (Elstein et al, 1978; Kassirer and Gorry, 1978) Instead, the experts' process is reported to be more like a shuttle between the patient's data field and the clinician's cerebral library of indexed, cross-referenced knowledge. The cues (usually pathognomonic cues or small clusters of cues) in the presenting situation lead clinicians to locate and retrieve packets of knowledge they have learned to link with these cues. These knowledge packets usually contain:

  a problem label or diagnostic classification,

  a list of characteristic features—risk factors, signs and symptoms, a statement of the parts of the body or systems involved and the underlying mechanisms producing the phenomenon, and

  a set of associated actions.

This mental shuttle is activated by surprisingly few cues. In one study age, sex, and a few cues on presenting complaints were enough to send the shuttle to the long-term memory library. (Kassirer and Gorry, 1978, p. 247) Other studies showed that this activation of provisional problem categories began for 95% of physicians and medical students within the first five minutes of the encounter. (Elstein et al, 1978, p. 168); Gordon, (1980) found similar immediate activation of multiple hypotheses in graduate nursing students. While traditional wisdom has taught the importance of reserving judgment until all the facts are in, why is it that outstanding practicing clinicians regularly function with such seeming prematurity in considering possible diagnoses?

Functions of Early Hypotheses Activation.   There seem to be two explanations for retrieving problem classifications early and trying them on for size. One has to do with reducing cognitive stress by increasing structure in the activity. The second deals with lending more efficient direction to subsequent data-search efforts.

The first explanation for seeking diagnostic possibilities early in the assessment encounter has to do with limiting the size of the search field and bringing it into manageable dimensions. Uncertainty, compounded by time constraints and expectations that the clinician will move expeditiously to an accurate decision, creates anxiety. That anxiety can be reduced by transforming open, nebulous search spaces into a series of tentatively closed provisional problem areas that can then be investigated sequentially or simultaneously. This gives a sense of structure and reduces cognitive strain.

The second feature of early hypothesis activation is that these hypotheses offer tentative terminal points plus directions for data search and interpretation. This again offers some security in structure that reduces anxiety and gives a sense of movement toward the expected goal of accurately defining the existing problem areas, ruling out others, and having a basis for initiating appropriate treatment.

The function of early hypothesizing, then, is in its adaptive value for selecting and managing information. It gives some structure and direction in a time-limited problem solving encounter.

Dangers of Early Hypothesis Activation.   The activation of hypotheses (early in the assessment encounter when cues taken in are, of necessity, still sparse and often ambiguous) is not without diagnostic dangers. Francis Bacon observed that once an opinion had been made, the mind tended to draw all things to support that judgment, ignoring the presence of contrary or ill-fitting data. In recent observation of physician diagnostic behavior, it was noted that, once hypotheses had been activated, nonconfirming data tended to be ignored. Such signals were seen as "noise" rather than stimuli to seek alternative possible explanations. (Elstein et al, 1978, p. 161)

Contrarily, it has also been found that many clinicians are loath to settle for the patient's initial presenting complaint as the major problem. All practicing clinicians have experienced the patients' opening gambits that are merely prologues to the real and perhaps more threatening problems that caused them to seek health care. For example, normotensive older persons often use a blood pressure check as the entree to geriatric nursing clinics when their real concerns are with other signs and symptoms that emerge tentatively and often much later in the assessment.

All this suggests that, while early hypotheses activation is a necessary part of diagnostic reasoning, the tentative nature of the hypotheses must be maintained. One cannot afford to fall in love with them. This is particularly crucial in nursing where the diagnostic focus has only recently emerged, the diagnostic concepts are fewer and less well-developed, the legitimacy of the nursing assessment-diagnostic behavior uncertain, and the time for this activity critically limited as pressures of non-diagnostic functions take precedence. There is every pressure to pick a diagnostic label, a familar one, and stay with it.

Being able to delimit problem areas and place diagnostic labels on them brings structure, closure, and a sense of accomplishment and comfort to the diagnostician. It reduces the sense of uncertainty and stress for the person charged with diagnostic responsibility. However, the temptation to become wedded to early diagnostic hypotheses and to seek that certainty prematurely is still to be avoided. The term "hypothesis" is deliberately chosen to maintain an open speculative stance while still offering some necessary structure and direction to assessments that have a compact time frame.

Short and Long Term Memory in Hypotheses Activation

Both short- and long-term memory are critical elements of the hypothesis activation–diagnostic sequence. Each must be understood as a resource if it is to be well used.

Short-Term Memory.   Short-term memory might be likened to a small busy control room during the initial patient encounter. Here the current transactions carried out include

holding limited quantities of data,

sending a retrieval shuttle to long-term memory stores
for associated knowledge,

combining the label-plus knowledge with the associated
data for short-term storage, and

directing subsequent observation maneuvers that are
derived from the knowledge–data combination.

The amount of information that can be held for working use in short-term memory is five to nine "chunks" (Simon, 1974, Mandler, 1967). Physicians who were studied fell within these norms as they were found using a maximum of four to six or seven, diagnostic possibilities during any stage of the workup. (Elstein et al, 1978; Wortman, 1972, p. 321)

A *chunk* of information is any stimulus that has become familiar through previous encounters so that it is recognizable as a single unit. (Larkin et al, 1980, p. 208; Simon, 1974). In the health care field, such chunks could be a single cue, cue clusters, or patterns of signs, symptoms and risk factors.

The difference between novices' and experts' abilities to deal with chunks of information involves several features. Novices' chunks tend to contain fewer elements and recognition is slower and more tentative. Experts' chunking encompasses more items within the recognized unit and recognition tends to be more rapid and secure. (Larkin et al, 1980; Tanner, Section 2).

This suggests that limitations imposed by short-term memory capacity of five to nine chunks can be expanded by the introduction of certain patterns in this chunking. Some strategies for enhancing the size of chunks, and thus the capacity of working information pools, include linking the data to diagnostic possibilities and structuring a relationship between diagnostic possibilities. The second type of strategy is a more mechanical one.

Developing *relationships between* hypotheses can assist in holding them available in short-term memory during the assessment-diagnostic process. Two strategies of placing hypotheses into explicit relationships are common—hierarchical and competing arrangements.

A *hierarchical relationship of general to specific* is useful because its organization allows for a more economical storage of cues. All available associated cues can be linked with the general diagnostic concept, while only selected ones will be associated with the more specific subcategories of the diagnosis. (Elstein et al, 1978, p. 180) Illustrations of this arrangement applied to both pathology and management of living domains will demonstrate the relationships. In management of daily living, as shown in the table below, the general diagnostic category of Loss may be associated with more specific hypotheses of Alienation/Loneliness, Grieving, Sensory Deprivation, or Immobilization.

Loss
Signs and symptoms: 1, 2, 3, 4, 5, 6, 7, 8
Risk factors: 1, 2, 3, 4

	Alienation/Loneliness	Grieving	Sensory Deprivation	Immobilization
Signs and Symptoms:	2, 3, 7	2, 6	4, 5, 8	1, 5, 7
Risk Factors:	1, 4	1	2, 3, 4	2

The same hierarchical arrangement in a pathophysiologic domain could be:

Gastrointestinal Disorder
Signs and Symptoms: 1, 2, 3, 4, 5, 6, 7, 8

Ulcerative Colitis	Intestinal Malignancy	Psychogenic Diarrhea
2, 3, 7	2, 6	1, 2, 5, 7

The general problem category develops a regional problem area and incorporates specific, more narrow problem spaces. The broader problem helps to avoid too narrow an approach to data collection. The specific hypotheses, on the other hand, help to ensure that cues of particular significance to a differential diagnosis are sought and interpreted. (Elstein et al, 1978, 180–181)

The second critical-thinking strategy for retaining hypotheses and data in a manageable number of chunks in short-term memory is to develop competing hypotheses and alternative explanations for the same phenomena. The use of competing hypotheses linked to each other enlarges the chunk size. It also serves to keep the diagnostician from becoming wedded to a possibly incorrect hypothesis too soon. (Kessel, 1969) A common situation in nursing is that a patient does not participate in a prescribed health behavior. Two competing diagnostic hypotheses are that he:

is unable to do it, physically or emotionally; CAN'T, or

does not wish to engage in the behavior; WON'T

The dynamics and treatment of "can't" (inability secondary to inadequate strength/endurance/knowledge/skill/courage) versus "won't" (lack of desire) are different. The entertaining of competing hypotheses may occur at both a general or specific level.

A mechanical strategy for holding cues available is, of course, the recording of them, in writing or otherwise, as the assessment is in progress. This is particularly critical for cues that don't seem to fit or cluster with the hypotheses that are being activated. Many experienced clinicians find that a recorded word or two will later reactivate remembrance of a large chunk of data they encountered with the patient during the assessment.

It is wise to be aware of the limitations of short-term memory and its implication for clinical judgments. It is also wise for the clinician to understand the strategies for expanding the size of chunks and to realize that this skill is a part of long-term professional growth.

Long-Term Memory.   Long-term memory may be likened to a very large indexed, cross referenced, and unindexed cerebral library in which knowledge, both factual (semantic) and experiential (episodic), is stored. Storage of information in long-term memory is thought to take seconds, while retrieval of accessible knowledge from long-term to short-term memory is achieved in milliseconds.

A great part of the professional clinician's education and ongoing growth is concerned with the acquisition, storage, and retrieval of basic and consistently updated knowledge, and the integration of clinical experience into semantic memory. When the knowledge and experience are deliberately stored with diagnostic strategies in mind, the access routes are also incorporated so that when particular cues (signs, symptoms, risk factors etc.) are perceived in the presenting situation, the appropriate packets of knowledge are retrieved. This means that the *indexing and cross referencing of the store of information* in terms of identifying features and associated action to permit retrieval upon encountering the cue pattern, *needs to be a conscious part of the storage process.*

A second major element in professional skill is gaining efficiency in using the access routes between the presenting situation and the packets of information in the long-term memory library. Expertise is achieved by repeated, extensive, critiqued experiences of encountering cues in varying circumstances and combinations and then retrieving the knowledge to classify and explain them. The development of speed and finesse in retrieving the most precise, relevant knowledge packets can become an element in the clinician's critical self analysis after any patient encounter, from either a pathophysiological or management of daily living perspective. One can note cues that were present and used, whether they were different from the previous recognition patterns or a reinforcement of those previously used. Such deliberate transfer of experience from purely episodic long-term memory to semantic memory can strengthen knowledge and recognition patterns.

Accuracy and speed in cue recognition and hypothesis activation are dependent upon the foundation of discipline-based content (semantic long-term memory) plus the stored previous experience with patient (episodic long-term memory), and upon using that content and developing access routes from cues in new situations to the knowledge experience packets.

Characteristics of Early Hypotheses.   The earliest hypotheses activated in the diagnostic sequence tend to be general in nature, as might be expected, and appropriate when the cues are still sparse and often ambiguous. For example, in a presenting situation of a person with chronic pain, hypothesis retrieval in the management of living domain could activate: sleep deprivation, immobilization, and alienation. These general hypotheses then create potential regional problem areas and lend direction for subsequent data search and more specific subdivision. Each of the contributors in Section 3 identifies the general hypotheses areas and the movement to more specific levels.

Logic versus Intuition in Hypothesis Activation.   Much of the literature deals with the diagnostic process in terms of objective, logical, scientific method, which indeed it is. Yet all practicing clinicians have diagnoses that pop into awareness without conscious logical effort. As noted on p. 29, this element of diagnostic reasoning has its place too, and since it is followed by further data-gathering to confirm or disconfirm, it can be as useful as diagnostic hypotheses generated in a more conscious fashion.

Summary

An early step in the process of organizing data for problem identification is to use the first recognized cues, though few and indefinite, to activate tentative diagnostic hypotheses that may explain what is being observed. Short-term memory, the cerebral vehicle for linking data to knowledge about it, can hold four to seven "chunks" of information for use. Such chunks can be made up of a cue, a cue cluster, or diagnostic hypotheses with their associated knowledge to link with the cues being held. Experience permits the clinician to develop and use larger, more complex chunks in short-term memory. Diagnostic hypotheses organized hierarchically, from general to specific or in competing formulations, have been found to be most useful in lending structure to subsequent data collection and interpretation. It is crucial to consider multiple explanatory hypotheses because of the ambiguity of early cues and the strong probability that multiple problems are coexisting.

Diagnostic hypothesis activation is often a conscious, logical, critical-thinking maneuver. However it can also occur without conscious effort, when diagnostic possibilities merely arise in one's awareness.

The packets of knowledge and experience that are drawn from long-term memory, either consciously or unconsciously in the hypothesis activating process, give structure and direction to subsequent assessment. This is accomplished as they:

delimit the data search spaces,

give direction to data collection by use of the profile of
problem manifestations (signs, symptoms, risk
factors),

offer tentative terminal points for clinical judgments.

The tentative nature of early hypotheses is important in order to avoid manipulating the data to fit an inaccurate or imprecise diagnosis. Subsequent cues that don't fit or that contradict early problem classifications challenge clinicians to consider other hypotheses—though research shows that there is a strong tendency for clinicians to ignore them.

This first step in using data effectively to generate explanations is a crucial one. Problem labels of diagnostic classifications that are not considered cannot be tested. Clinicians make right diagnoses because they think of them. The ultimate success as well as the efficiency of the remainder of the assessment-diagnostic process rests on the quality of this initial and recurring step in the process.

Hypothesis Evaluation

Where the first stage in the problem identification process is concerned with generating a number of possible classifications to explain the findings in the presenting situation, the next stage concerns itself with a refining or revising of these possibilities. The first involves divergent thinking; the latter convergent thinking.

The diagnostic concepts drawn from long-term memory offer a profile of features associated with that particular problem classification. These frequently include:

antecedent events,

risk factors that increase the likelihood of the problem
occurring,

prevalence of the problem,

patterns of events or manifestations associated with the
development of the problem,

signs and symptoms indicating the problem's presence
and stage of development,

underlying mechanisms involved in the problem and
relationships to other systems,

complications,

variables affecting outcome (prognosis),

responsiveness to treatment,

activities associated with effective management of the
problem, and

criteria for evaluating response to treatment and course
of the problem.

The knowledge and experience associated with the first five components are the ones that offer the most direction in the data search for
diagnoses, although in some disciplines the responsiveness to treatment is used to set priority of attention.

Refinement of the problem classification consists of searching
the data field for cues associated with the features of the problems
being considered and matching them with the problem profiles for
congruence or goodness of fit. Where competing alternative hypotheses have been activated, it is possible to match the presenting data
against each profile and determine where the fit is most congruent.
Where both general and specific hypotheses have been retained, the
data usually permits movement toward one of the more specific diagnoses.

If data are present or arise in later stages of the assessment that
do not fit the initial hypotheses, new hypotheses must be generated
and the process repeated. As the hypothesis evaluation progresses,
earlier diagnostic possibilities are rejected or refined to specify this
particular person's situation at this time.

The final stage of this hypotheses evaluation process is to select
a diagnostic classification as precise as the available data will permit.
This choice in classification (diagnosis) plus the data become the
foundation for decisions about prognosis, goals, and treatment plans
and activities.

Definitive Diagnosis.   The final stage in making a clinical judgment about the nature of the presenting health problems is that of
assigning to them the most precise labels appropriate, given the available data. They are the end product of hypothesis activation and
evaluation. Reaching this point has involved moving from general
problem areas to specific ones or choosing among competing specific
hypotheses.

The components usually included in a definitive diagnostic statement show interesting parallels between the pathophysiologic model and the management of the daily model, as seen in the following table.

Pathophysiologic Diagnosis	Management of Daily Living Diagnosis
Target organ or system	Target areas of daily living affecting/affected by health status
Pathologic process	Inadequate or decreasing internal and/or external resources
Causative agent	Situation depleting or demanding new use of internal and/or external resources
Time element (acute/chronic)	Same

For example, a pathophysiologic diagnosis would be *Osteoporotic fracture of right hip,* while a parallel management of daily living diagnosis would be, *Usual high independence and return to former solo lifestyle threatened by fractured hip high anxiety.*

General problem labels have two major uses. They are necessary, at times, in initial stages of diagnosis. They are also useful in designating categories of problems for statistical purposes. A general diagnosis, however, is not adequate as a basis for prescribing treatment from either perspective. Effective treatment of pathology cannot be mounted with a diagnosis of neoplasm or infection. Nor can effective treatment in management of daily living problems be developed from diagnoses such as immobilization or sensory deprivation. For predictably useful treatment to occur, a specific diagnosis of this individual's problem at this time is essential.

Prognosis

Once the problem label has been made as specific as the data and knowledge about the phenomenon allow, there is one more clinical judgment to be made prior to making decisions about treatment. A prognostic judgment must be made and taken into account as a basis for setting up the treatment plan.

Prognosis is a statement predicting trajectory and outcome. Vocabulary associated with prognosis includes: cure, stable, recovered, progressive, end stage, terminal, acute, chronic, remission, exacerbation, cyclic, short/long term and so on.

As in the process of arriving at a diagnosis, the judgments in making a prognostic statement derive from both knowledge of the phenomena involved and data from the patient and his situation. Where pathology is the focus, this most frequently involves understanding the pathology and its effects, the usual course of the disease or event, the effect of risk factors, and those that affect responsiveness to treatment. The person who is host to the pathology or changed health status also presents variables in terms of age, genetic heritage, general health (past and present), risk factors, resources, and environment, all of which are incorporated into the prediction of the likely course of events.

Where the focus is management of daily living, the same process occurs as consideration is given to variables affecting the likelihood of success and satisfaction in managing daily living with presenting health problems or issues. This perspective too requires integration of both knowledge and data in several areas:

- □ the status of internal and external resources
- □ the nature of demands being placed on them (pathology, treatment, present, future)
- □ the predicted course of events for the health problem and the implications for future functioning activities and demands of daily living, use of external resources, and changing relationships with the environment within which that living takes place

Just as specificity in diagnosis is needed for effective treatment decisions, so are sound judgments regarding prognosis. All of the elements of the prognosis—course of events, duration, and outcome—influence treatment choices in any health care discipline.

Decisions on Treatment.   Once the diagnosis has been made as precise as possible and the prognosis has been reviewed, choices of treatment options and priorities can then be considered and decisions can be made. In the health care fields, management decisions constitute plans for deliberate intervention on the part of the care provider to influence the course of events in a designated problem area. The care provider may prescribe activities to try to :

retain wellness,

prevent, delay or minimize health problems at risk,

interfere with the normal dynamics and progress of the health problem so as to shorten it, reduce intensity or remove it,

prevent complications and additional treatment-related (iatrogenic) problems,

minimize the negative effects of chronic problems and
those that cause growing dysfunction and threat to
life.

The kinds of intervention that health care providers in any discipline
will consider or be prepared to consider and undertake are influenced
by several factors. These include: discipline specific to training, tradition, and, in some cases, the law.

As in all the other steps of the diagnostic-management decision
pattern, both knowledge and data are integrated into decisions regarding treatment. The knowledge involved in treatment decisions
requires an understanding of the underlying mechanisms associated
with the phenomenon, such as pathology, psychosocial dynamics,
and the dynamics of interaction between the elements of stressors
and host. Beyond this in some disciplines, such as nursing, the relationship of the person and his associated health status to his lifestyle
and environment is another component to be incorporated when arriving at judicious management decisions.

The nature and extent of health-care-provider intervention
ranges widely. The decision may be to:

do nothing,

give information so the client or family can make
decisions regarding *self care,*

recommend (mildly or strongly) a pattern of self-care or
a decision to seek professional help,

obtain informed consent for specified activity by the
professional,

assume the right of making the patient's decision for him
and require professional care, determining both the
nature and location of that care,

engage in explicit physical and/or interpersonal activities,
undertaken to alter the problem and the patient's
response to it, or to

engage in activities to modify the environment, including
the availability and use of external resources.

Concurrently with the decisions of whether and how to inter-
vene comes the decision of sequence of prescribed behavior and the
urgency for taking action. Decisions regarding the *timing* of professionals' activities can be as crucial as any other dimension of the
diagnostic management sequence. Some interventions are so ur-
gently required that, if delayed, they are useless. An obvious example
of this are the measures to treat cardiac arrest or respiratory obstruction. Other activities, to be useful, must be timed to occur before

particular events, such as contraception prior to sexual activity, or preparation to participate in health-related behaviors such as infant care or diagnostic tests or treatments. On the other hand, treatment that is introduced prematurely can also be ineffective. Pushing for explicit acceptance of a changed body status when the person is still in a normal and useful denial stage, teaching before the person is ready to learn, or encouraging exercise while a myocardial infarction lesion has not reached an appropriate healing stage are all examples of premature intervention. For professional treatment to be effective the decisions regarding timing of activities are critical.

Evaluation and Revision

Life is a dynamic and transient state. Health problems and host responses are rarely static and are often unpredictable. Therefore, ongoing clinical judgments regarding the person's status and response to treatment are another important step in the judgment-decision pattern. These include continuing review of the status of previously diagnosed problems and risk areas as well as scanning of the person's current situation afresh for changes, in each subsequent encounter.

Intervals for Monitoring.   It should be noted that the intervals between planned periods of monitoring are important decision areas also. These encounters can be so frequent that they become not only overly expensive, but they also generate fear in the person. At the other extreme, they could be so infrequent as to miss changes that should receive early treatment. The assessments in ongoing encounters with the clientele are similar to the patterns used in the original assessment.

Variables for Evaluation.   In addition to these decisions, the health care provider is concerned with evaluating the response to the treatment that actually has been undertaken. How have the problem dynamics and/or host responses been changed by the intervention? Is it in the desired direction? Are any side effects also occurring? Is the original prognosis still holding? Given the nature of the response, should current protocols be continued? If not, what revisions should be made? What risk factors have changed? Are support systems holding?

In the evaluation and revision stages it is obvious that the entire initial pattern is repeated with the change that more longitudinal data plus new data are available and interventions by one or more elements of the health care system have been introduced.

SUMMARY

The patterns of interaction between client data and discipline knowledge to produce clinical judgments and decisions are comparable across all health professions. Variation comes in the discipline-specific perspective taken in viewing the situation, the body of knowledge commonly drawn upon, the problem-classification system (taxonomy), the focus of prognosis with its associated variables, and the treatment options available to practitioners in that profession.

Nurses, both because of tradition and patients' needs, regularly direct their clinical judgments and decision making to determining when the patients' presenting situation requires the judgments and decisions to be made in each discipline and which should be addressed first.

Nurses have been biased by both tradition and training to direct the process primarily and explicitly to the medical field, even when medical personnel have been available or have already engaged in this activity. The third section of this book will demonstrate the patterns nursing clinicians are using to address the process of making clinical judgments and decisions in the nursing domain. As nurses see examples of how it can be done, it is hoped that more will make appropriate and cost-effective choices as to when to direct their judgments and decisions to the management of daily living as this relates to health, and when to address primarily the person's health status.

BIBLIOGRAPHY

Annual Conference on Research in Medical Education. (entire issue) Nov, 1979

Aspinall MJ, Tanner C: Decision Making for Patient Care, Applying the Nursing Process. New York, Appleton–Century–Crofts, 1981

Aspinall, MJ: Use of a decision tree to improve accuracy of diagnosis, Nursing Research 28:182–185, May–June 1979

Berne E: Intuition and Ego States. San Francisco, Transactional Publications, 1977

Biörck G: The essence of the clinician's art. Acta Med Scand 201:145–147, 1977

Broderick, Mary and William Ammentorp: Information structures: an analysis of nursing performance. Nursing Research: 28:106–110, March–April 1979

Copeland D: Concepts of disease and diagnosis. Perspect Biol Med Summer, 1977

de Dombal FT: Medical diagnosis from a clinician's point of view. Methods Inf Med 17:28–35, 1978

Denham J: Educational obstacles to learning diagnosis. J Fam Pract 12, No. 4:665–669, 1981

Dykes M: Uncritical thinking in medicine. J Amer Med Asso 227:1275–1277, 1974

Elstein A: Clinical judgment: psychological research and medical practice. Science 194:698–700, 1976

Elstein A, Shulman L, Sprafka S: Medical Problem Solving: An Analysis of Clinical Reasoning. Cambridge, Harvard University Press, 1978

Feinstein AR: Clinical judgment. Baltimore, Williams and Wilkins, 1967

Gale J: Some cognitive components of the diagnostic thinking process. Br. J Ed Psych 52 (*Pt. 1*) 64–76, February 1982

Gordon M et al: Nursing diagnosis: looking at its use in the clinical area. Am J of Nurs 80:672–74, 1980

Gordon M: Predictive strategies in diagnostic task. Nursing Research 29:39–45, Jan–Feb, 1980

Gordon M: Nursing Diagnosis, Process and Application. New York, Mc-Graw-Hill, 1982

Hammond KR, McClelland GH and Mumpower J: Human judgment and decision making, New York, Praeger, 1980

Harris JM: The hazards of bedside Bayes JAMA, 246(22) 2602-5 Dec. 4, 1981

Jaquez JA (ed): The diagnostic process. Pro Conf, University of Michigan, Ann Arbor, 1964

Kassirer J and Gorry GA: Clinical problem solving behavior. Annals of Internal Medicine 89:245–255, August, 1978

Kern L et al: Pseudodiagnosticity in an idealized medical problem solving environment. J of Med Educ 57(2) 100–104, February 1982

Kessel FS: The philosophy of science as proclaimed and science as practiced: identity or dualism. Amer Psychol 24:999–1005, 1969

Kreel L et al: The diagnostic process: a comparison of scanning techniques. Br Med J, 2:809–811, Sept 24, 1977

Larkin, Jill et al: Expert and Novice performance in solving physics problems. Science 208:1335–1342, June 20, 1980

Ledley R and Husted LB: Reasoning foundations of medical diagnosis. Science 130:9–21, July 1959

Leaper DJ et al: Clinical diagnostic process: an analysis. B Med J, 2:569–571, Sept 15, 1973

Lusted LB: Introduction to Medical Decision Making. Springfield, Illinois, CC Thomas, 1968

Mandler GA: Organization and memory. In Spencer JT (eds): The Psychology of Learning and Motivation Vol 1, New York, Academic Press, 1967

Matthews, CA and Gaul AL: Nursing Diagnosis from the perspective of concept attainment and critical thinking. *Advances in Nursing* Science 2, 1:17–26, October 1979

McGaghie WC: Medical Problem-Solving: a reanalysis, J Med Ed 55:912–921, 1980

Meehl PE: The cognitive activity of the clinician. Am. Psychol, 15:19–27, 1960

Miller GA: The magical number seven, plus or minus two: Some limits to our capacity for processing information. Psychol Rev 63:81–97, 1956

Mynatt CR et al: Consequences of confirmation and disconfirmation in a simulated research environment. Q J Exp Psychol 30:395–406, 1978

Newell An, Simon HA: Human Problem Solving. Englewood Cliffs, New Jersey, Prentice Hall, 1972

Nurs Clin North Am (entire issue), March, 1979

Palton D: Introduction to clinical decision making. Semin Nucl Med 8, No. 4:273–282, Oct. 1978

Pauker SG, Kassirer JP: Clinical application of decision analysis. Semin Nucl Med 8, No. 4:324–325, Oct, 1978

Popper KR: The Logic of Scientific Discovery. New York, Basic Books, 1959

Price RB, Vlahcevic ZK: Logical principles in differential diagnosis. Ann Intern Med 75:89–95, 1971

Rosenhan DL: On being sane in insane places. Science 179:250–258, Jan. 1973

Schwartz WB et al: Decision analysis and clinical judgment. Amer J Med 55:459–472, 1973

Simon H: How big is a chunk? Science 183:482–488, Feb 8, 1974

Style A: Intuition and problem solving. Journal of Royal College of General Practice 199:71–74, Feb 1979

Tanner CA: Instruction on the diagnostic process: an experimental study in Kim MJ, and Moritz DA (eds): Classification of Nursing Diagnoses, pp 145–152, New York, McGraw-Hill 1982

Tversky A: Judgment under uncertainty: Heuristics and biases. Science 185:1124–1131, 1974

Wortman P: Medical diagnosis: an information processing approach. Comput Biomed Res 5:315–328, 1972

Pre-encounter Influences on Data Gathering and Interpretation

Adebimpe VR: Overview: white norms and psychiatric diagnosis of black patients. Amer J Psychiatry 138:279–285, Mar, 1981

Armitage KJ et al: Response of physicians to medical complaints of men and women. J Amer Med Assoc 241, No. 20:2186–2187, 1979

Coles R: A fashionable kind of slander. Atlantic Monthly, 226:53–55, 1970

Ehrenreich B: Gender and objectivity in medicine. Int Health Serv 4, No. 4:617–623, 1974

Eisenberg JM: Sociologic influences on decision making by clinicians. Ann Intern Med 90, No. 6:957–964, 1979

Fidell LS: Sex role stereotypes and the American physician. Psychol Wom Q 4, No. 3:313–330, 1980

Fielding G et al: An exploratory experimental study of the influence of patients' social background upon the diagnostic process and outcomes. Psychiatr Clin 11, No. 2:61–86, 1978

Howell MC: What medical schools teach about women. N Engl J Med 291:304–307, 1974

Kraus VL: Pre-information—its effects on nurses' descriptions of a patient. J Nurs Ed 15:18–26, 1976

Scheff TJ: Typification in the diagnostic practice of rehabilitation. pp 139–143.

In N. Sussman, ed. Sociology and Rehabilitation. American Sociologic Assoc. 1965

Suchman EA: Social patterns of illness and medical care. J Health Hum Behav 6, No. 1:2–16, 1965

Verbrugge LM: Sex differences in complaints and diagnoses. J Behav Med 3, No. 4:327–355, 1980

Wallen J et al: Physician stereotypes about female health and illness: a study of patients' sex and the information process during medical interviews Women and Health, 4, No. 2:135–146, 1979

Stages of Development in Diagnostic Expertise: Characteristics, Constraints, and Strategies

Christine A. Tanner

Toward the Development of Diagnostic Reasoning Skills

Students of the health sciences typically are taught the classical scientific method of problem solving. They are taught to systematically accumulate all the data, proceed with an unprejudiced analysis of the data—withholding judgment until the facts are in—and derive a logical conclusion about the meaning of the data. Having learned this process, the students, who have spent hours questioning and requestioning the client, poring over records, and comparing data with textbook descriptions, are often struck by the seeming ease with which experienced diagnosticians derive a probable diagnosis, using very little data and a few directed questions. What may seem like an intuitive leap for the expert is really *another* systematic process that proceeds along lines quite dissimilar to those embodied in the classical empiricist approach.

The reason expert diagnosticians have adopted an alternative process to the scientific method is clear. Humans have limited information-processing capabilities; they simply do not have the storage capacity in short-term memory to perform all of the mental gymnastics required in a diagnostic task using the classical method. The

57

alternative process is composed of a set of reliable strategies which allow diagnosticians to make the most of their limited processing capabilities in short-term memory and to use, to the fullest extent, the massive storehouse of knowledge in long-term memory.

This is not to say that the student or novice diagnostician cannot make sound clinical judgments or engage in appropriate clinical activities. Indeed, the scientific method has withstood the test of time; the practice of systematic data collection and analysis is an important activity in any clinical problem-solving task. However, there is a natural human tendency among diagnosticians, particularly when faced with the time constraints of clinical practice, to try and fit the problem-solving task to the limitations imposed by information processing capabilities. Hence, even the novice begins to adopt some of the same cognitive strategies employed by the experts in making a clinical judgment. The adoption of such strategies may occur at the preconscious level, so that the diagnostician may be unaware of the extent to which their use may have influenced the decision made.

The purpose of this section is to make explicit the cognitive strategies used by both the novice and the expert in making clinical judgments, and to look at the implications of these patterns of critical thinking. In Chapter 3, we examine the factors that influence the diagnostic process, including both the characteristics of diagnostic tasks and the capabilities of the human information processing system. In Chapter 4, we explore the cognitive strategies used by novices and experts to make the most of their mental powers when faced with complex diagnostic tasks.

The ideas presented in this section are drawn from a rapidly expanding body of research designed for the investigation of diagnostic processes used by physicians, medical students, and (to a lesser extent) psychologists, nurses, and nursing students. The underlying assumption is that, while the domain of clinical decision-making differs across disciplines, the cognitive processes are essentially the same. Many of the examples of patient situations and nurses' responses to them are drawn from a study currently in progress.*

The purpose of the study is to examine the diagnostic reasoning strategies used by beginning, mid-level and experienced nurses. The data from the study have not been fully analyzed, so the interpretations offered, although based on extant cognitive theory, are inevita-

* Tanner CA, Putzier DJ, Westfall U and Padrick K: "Diagnostic Reasoning: An Analysis of Cognitive Strategies Used by Nursing Students and Nurses." Study in progress funded by Northwest Area Foundation Grant to Oregon Health Sciences University, 1982

bly incomplete. In fact, as we complete our analysis of all subjects' performances, it is possible that quite different interpretations will be appropriate. Where there is no scientific evidence of expert or novice performances in certain components of the diagnostic process, conjectures about probable performances are offered. It is with some "dis-ease," or more accurately, fear and trepidation, that these possibilities are offered, because they may not hold up under scientific scrutiny, or more importantly, that once into print, they will be interpreted as law. The reader is asked to use her best critical judgment in assessing the extent to which the suggestions of this section fit with reality.

CHAPTER THREE

Factors Influencing the Diagnostic Process

Christine A. Tanner

The way all humans think, and specifically the way they tackle problems, is a function of two major factors: (1) the characteristics of problem-solvers—notably how much information they can process from the environment and how well they can remember information stored in memory; and (2) the characteristics of the problem and how the problem-solver perceives those characteristics. The cognitive strategies used in diagnostic reasoning represent the ways the clinicians have adapted their own limited information-processing resources to the demands of the problem.

As an example, consider the following situation: Mrs. Young is a 50-year-old patient with myasthenia gravis. She was hospitalized two weeks ago with myasthenia crisis, which required tube-feeding and frequent nasopharyngeal-suctioning. She regained strength, apparently moved to remission, and was transferred from the critical-care unit to a general-medical unit two days ago. During the evening and night shift, she has been turning on her call light frequently, requesting assistance in turning, reaching a glass of water, and so on, even though she is now capable of doing those things herself. The following is a report provided by an expert nurse on how she handled the situation:

> The nurse aide complained to me that Mrs. Young had been on her light all night long. Her whining and always asking what time it was were driving the aide crazy. For some reason, I cued in on Mrs. Young always asking about the time. I know that if myasthenia patients don't get their prostigmine right on time, they begin to develop muscle weakness and can quickly get into trouble. I talked this over with Mrs. Young and she

confirmed that she was scared about the possibility of another crisis and just hated to be alone. We worked out a system in which she could take her own medications. Mrs. Young felt like she could be in control of taking her own meds.

This nurse could not have taken appropriate action based only on the cues presented by Mrs. Young; the demanding behavior was perceived by the nurse as being symptomatic of a more basic problem. She used her knowledge of human behavior, coupled with her understanding of the disease process, to make an *inference* about the meaning of the cues. While the situation held a potentially infinite amount of data that the nurse might have collected, she focused her attention on what seemed to be the most likely explanation for Mrs. Young's behavior. She sought the most reliable data (in this case, discussing her inference with Mrs. Young) in order to confirm or rule out the diagnosis. In this way, she efficiently derived the diagnosis: *fear of repeated myasthenia crisis related to lack of control over medication administration.*

Although the nurse could not explicitly explain why she had approached the problem the way she did, it is likely that the strategies she adopted were governed by at least two factors. First, at some level, the nurse recognized that the behavior was symptomatic of another more basic problem. Stated another way, she recognized that there was a *a probabilistic relationship between the cue and the diagnosis.* She obtained additional data to reduce the uncertainty in making her inference. Secondly, she used a strategy to reduce cognitive strain; by focusing her attention on the most likely explanation for the behavior, she conserved her limited information-processing resources.

In this chapter, we explore in greater depth both the characteristics of the task environment in diagnosis and the information-processing resources that typify the human problem-solver. We will also examine the interaction between these two factors, and the differences that are likely to exist between the novice and expert diagnostician.

TASK CHARACTERISTICS

Diagnostic tasks are characterized by uncertain and probabilistic relationships between cues (signs and symptoms) and the internal state(s) of the patient. *The act of diagnosis is the process of inferring the unobservable state of the client from uncertain, observable data presented by the client.* It is this probabilistic nature of the relationship between cues and the internal state of the client which make the inference process so complex.

Probabilities

We frequently make statements using words like "all", "some", and "no," as in "All patients prior to surgery experience anxiety," or "Some patients have less preoperative anxiety after teaching." Statements such as these are really expressions of probability or proportion and can be described mathematically. For example, one might express the first statement as "Patient X has a 100% probability of experiencing preoperative anxiety". "With teaching, Patient X has a 50% chance of having his anxiety reduced".

The use of probability statements is commonplace in medicine. On informed consents for medical procedures, for example, many states require that the probability of complications be explicitly stated, *e.g.*, the chance of developing a blood clot after an arteriogram is 5%. Generally such probability statements are derived from repeated and systematic observations on a large sample of individuals.

In the health sciences, probabilities are more commonly expressed as conditional probabilities. If A is present, then B follows. For example, *if* a patient is immobile, *then* there is a chance for decubitus-ulcer formation. *If* the patient is immobile, and *if* the patient is elderly, and *if* the patient's nutritional status is poor, *then* the probability of decubitus is 95%.

One might well argue that the notion of probabilities, especially their mathematical expressions, is a meaningless exercise in nursing-clinical judgments. It is true that probability statements are best derived from systematic observations of a large group of individuals. And it is also true that we lack sufficient empirical base in nursing for precise expression of probabilistic relations. Yet students of clinical decision-making argue that both diagnosis and prognosis rest on at least the informal assignment of probabilities to clinical data. Failure to recognize the probabilistic relationship between cues and client states leads to errors in diagnosis.

Use of Probabilities in Diagnosis

Let us look at an example of diagnosis from the biomedical domain. Nursing students learn that signs and symptoms of hypoglycemia, secondary to short-acting insulin, include a change in behavior, irritability, tremulousness, cold and clammy skin, and diaphoresis. They also learn that the causes of hypoglycemic reaction are delayed or omitted meals, excessive exercise, or insulin overdosage.

If a diabetic patient displays a change in behavior, the nurse, based on her knowledge, would entertain the diagnostic hypothesis of hypoglycemic reaction. The cue, *behavior change*, indicates insulin reaction, but in the absence of other data, other diagnoses may share the same probability. The nurse must accumulate other cues, each with some probabilistic relationship to the hypothesis of hypoglycemic reaction. If the behavior change is classified as irritability, the probability of hypoglycemic reaction increases. If the patient is diaphoretic and tremulous, the probability further increases. The nurse would also explore other causal relationships; if it was also found that the patient had omitted a meal, then the inference of hypoglycemic reaction would be almost certain. Note that the *diagnosis is confirmed through accumulation of data and informally revising the probability of the hypothesis with each datum.* A blood sugar is the only cue that might bear a positive relationship to hypoglycemia of sufficient magnitude that no other data would be needed.

Two important points are illustrated in this example. First, diagnostic tasks possess the characteristic of uncertainty; this uncertainty is created by the less-than-perfect relationship between any given cue and the state of the client. The uncertainty is reduced by accumulating data, with each positive cue increasing the probability of the hypothesized diagnosis. **Recognition of the probabilistic relationship between cues and diagnosis increases the thoroughness of data collection and improves diagnostic accuracy.**

Secondly, and perhaps less apparently, the kind of data typically available to the nurse for judgments both in the biomedical domain and (especially) in the nursing domain, is often unreliable. Nurses must rely almost entirely on their own perceptual processes; the more precise instruments used by physicians for medical decisions are not typically available or useful for nursing decisions. In this sense, the nurse's task is cognitively complex, for the effect of greater precision through instrumentation is to reduce the uncertainty and remove the need for accumulating numerous data.

Let's consider an example of a diagnosis-gone-wrong, tracing its origins to a faulty assignment of probability. A nursing student encountered the following situation: Mrs. Jamison is a 63-year-old widow recovering from coronary artery bypass surgery. She is 14 days post-op and plans are being made for her discharge. The student is assisting Mrs. Jamison to prepare for her noontime meal. Mrs. Jamison states that she feels weak and is unable to eat. She asks that the student help her sit up and she is barely able to pick up her fork. She says, "I feel so tired. I just don't think I'm ready to go home. Would you help me put my robe on?" Mrs. Jamison later complains of a burning pain in the epigastric area.

The following is what the student described as her thinking about Mrs. Jamison's situation:

> She has massive dependency needs. She seems to
> be really wanting everybody to do things for her. I don't
> think that's very good. I don't know for sure, but it
> seems like 14 days post-op she should be doing more for
> herself. I think I'd want to sit down with her and have a
> long talk with her about her anxiety. She doesn't want to
> go home. I mean she says that very clearly. Probably
> because she doesn't want to go home, she might blow
> up any kind of pain that she might have as being a very
> monumental thing. She's gonna have a hard time at
> home.

The student proceeded to get more information about Mrs. Jamison's home situation. She found on the chart that Mrs. Jamison lives in a mobile home with her sister. She continued with her inferences: "Well, I'd worry a lot about how she's gonna manage at home. They won't be able to afford much and if she's on a special diet, she'll have more difficulties."

Two major errors are apparent in this situation. First, the student did not recognize the probabilistic relationship between the cues (requesting assistance, complaints of weakness) and dependency. In fact, "massive dependency needs" had low probability, while the weakness may well have had a physiological origin. The probability of concern about going home was higher, and the student did indeed seek some additional data to discover the etiology of that concern.

The second error was the inference drawn about financial status and the general diagnosis of difficulty coping based on that inference. The student, when questioned, explained:

> I figured that they weren't too well-off because they
> lived in a trailer. Most people who live in trailers don't
> have much income. Her sister probably has to work and
> there won't be anyone to care for Mrs. Jamison when
> she goes home.

In making this inference, the student assigned a high conditional probability to the relationship, "*if* living in a mobile home, *then* low income." Further inferences were derived from the presumed financial status—the need for the sister to work and therefore, the unavailability of anyone to care for Mrs. Jamison. The result was a diagnosis not founded in fact.

To summarize, the recognition of the probabilistic relationship between cues and internal states of the client greatly influence the diagnostic process. Specifically, the kind of data obtained, as well as the amount of data obtained, will be influenced by the clinician's ability to informally assign conditional probabilities to a hypothesized diagnosis and to revise the probabilities in light of new data. The complexity of the diagnostic task is, in part, determined by the reliability of the data and the strength of the relationship between cues and states of the client. Several other factors influence task complexity. These factors are discussed in the following section.

Diagnostic Task Complexity

In a thoughtful analysis of inferences in nursing, Hammond (1966) described three kinds of diagnostic tasks: (1) determining the presence or absence of an 'abnormal state' based on the presence or absence of a single cue, (2) determining the presence or absence of an 'abnormal state' based on many cues, and (3) differentiating between two or more 'abnormal states' on the basis of many cues. The complexity of each of these tasks increases exponentially with the addition of cues and the number of potential client states. Rarely in the nursing situation can a diagnosis be reduced to a simple 'present' or 'absent' decision. If a client is presenting several cues, then the task is one of finding the diagnosis that best explains the majority of the cues. This typically is represented in a differential diagnosis in which two or more competing explanations are weighed against the probability of multiple cues. Because of the probability relations involved, an enormous cognitive burden is placed on the clinician. The greater the cognitive burden, the more crucial it is for the clinician to adopt strategies which make most efficient use of limited information-processing capabilities.

In addition to the specific characteristics of the diagnostic tasks, the cues possess a number of characteristics which greatly influence the complexity of diagnosis, the cognitive strain imposed, and the resulting strategies adopted to reduce the strain.

Number of cues: the greater the number of cues
   presented, the more complex the task.
Dependability: some cues are nearly infallible indicators
   of certain client states while others have low
   probability of occurrence. The greater the
   dependability of the available cues, the fewer the cues
   needed and the less the cognitive strain.

Redundancy: this term refers to the amount of repetitive information in a message. When a given state of the client exhibits two cues which always occur at the same time, then redundancy is said to be perfect. In general, the greater the redundancy, the easier the task; the information provided by the cues is, in essence, repeated, so it increases the certainty of the diagnosis.

Overlapping cues: in cases where there are two or more possible client states, there are some cues that are dependable indicators of all the possible states. For example, the patient who expressed concern about going home could have been exhibiting a cue related to physical weakness and, in turn, a physiological problem; or the cue may have been related to a nonsupportive home environment. The extent to which cues are overlapping in differential diagnosis influences the degree of task complexity.

Irreducible uncertainty: some diagnostic tasks have some degree of uncertainty which cannot be removed. As Hammond (1966, p. 35) points out, in these tasks ". . . no greater amount of clear thinking, no more careful logic, no further information and no greater medical knowledge will reduce the uncertainty." This situation is not uncommon in nursing and creates quite a dilemma for the clinician who is fearful of acting before all uncertainty is removed.

Recognition of factors influencing the complexity of clinical inference tasks is crucial for successful diagnosis. There exists a pervasive human tendency to try to simplify our environment. For example, holding stereotypes about groups of people allows us to codify and categorize our perceptions and to respond with a limited degree of taxing thought. Expert clinicians are those who recognize the fallibility of the cues they obtain, identify the multiplicity of cues available, capitalize on redundant information and realize when the uncertainty can no longer be reduced.

CHARACTERISTICS OF THE DIAGNOSTICIAN

Much of the research on diagnostic reasoning has its foundations in information processing theory (Newell & Simon, 1972; Simon, 1978). The theory likens the human mind to a computer and concerns itself with the interaction between the information-processing system (the problem-solver) and the demands of the task environment. We have seen from our previous discussion that the task environment in diagnosis is tremendously complex and holds the potential for placing a huge cognitive burden on the problem-solver. The major assumption underlying this theory is that there are limits to human information-processing capacity. Effective problem-solving, including diagnosis, rests on the system's ability to adapt to these limitations and to thereby reduce the cognitive strain imposed by the task.

Two types of limitations are critical: 1) factors that determine the amount of information to which the human can attend, and 2) factors that determine the clarity and accessibility of information internal to the problem-solver (*e.g.*, the ability to remember clearly the meaning of clinical data). These limitations are imposed by the structure and capacity of the two main memory systems—short-term memory (STM) and long-term memory (LTM).

Short-Term Memory

The short-term memory (STM) is our working memory. It is the active part of the mind where all incoming information from the environment is processed with knowledge drawn from long-term memory (LTM). Once information is processed in STM it is either forgotten or shuttled back for storage in the LTM.

One characteristic of the STM is its short duration (hence, the name short-term). Information in STM lasts only about 30 seconds unless it is actively processed through such activities as rehearsal. New information entering STM causes previously entered information to be lost. We've all had the experience of looking up a telephone number, saying it over and over (rehearsing it) to help us remember, only to be interrupted before we can place the call and quickly forgetting the number.

Another characteristic of the STM is its small capacity. Miller (1956) reported that the STM holds an invariant number of symbols (7 ± 2) but the capacity can be dramatically increased by coding familiar stimulus patterns into single units. A simple exercise will clarify this point. Two lists of words will be presented. Read the first list, one word every few seconds, close the book and attempt to recall the list:

PINE
DOCTOR
HOUSE

OAK
POTATO
CHURCH
LAWYER
SCHOOL
BROCCOLI
STORE
MAPLE
TEACHER
PEAS
ELM
SECRETARY
CARROTS

The words on the list fall into four categories: trees, buildings, occupations, and vegetables. They were presented in a disorganized manner and it is unlikely that you were able to remember more than seven of the words. Each of the words represents one unit of information or a total of 16—well beyond the capacity of STM.

Let's try another list, organized differently. After reading the list, at the same rate as the first, close your book and try to recall it:

LAWNMOWER
RAKE
SHOVEL
SPADE
TENNIS
SKIING
SWIMMING
RUNNING
ORANGES
APPLES
BANANAS
PEARS
DOGS
CATS
BIRDS
MICE

This time you should have been able to recall more of the words on the list, if you considered first the category label (for example, lawn tools, sports, fruits, and animals). The list could be even more efficiently recalled if you developed subcategories. For example, under the sports category, two are considered aerobic and two are not.

The list of animals could be recalled if you think of dogs chasing cats, cats chasing birds, and birds chasing mice.

So how does all this apply to diagnosis? In the first section of this chapter, we noted that diagnostic tasks are characterized by a huge amount of data, which have some probabilistic relationship to possible states of the client. If the data were not organized in some fashion as it enters STM it would quickly be forgotten. Categorizing the cues with respect to diagnostic hypotheses is one way the capacity of STM can be dramatically increased, and the limited information-processing resources conserved.

The categories for classifying information are retrieved from long-term memory. For example, the labels used to define the categories in the lists above are stored in LTM; the categories were used to coalesce the words into a smaller number of units. The organization of LTM, then, clearly influences the individual's capacity to conserve space in STM.

Long-Term Memory

The LTM is roughly composed of two types of memory systems (Klatzky, 1975). *Episodic* memory stores information about significant episodes in one's life—autobiographical information like "I graduated from college in 1975." Also stored in this memory is information about particular patient situations that have been encountered—the favorite patient, the most unusual patient, what happened the last time this presenting situation occurred. *Semantic* memory, on the other hand, holds information such as rules of English grammar, rules for adding and subtracting, and biomedical and nursing knowledge.

In addition to differences in what they store, semantic and episodic memory also differ in their susceptibility to forgetting. Information in episodic memory can become inaccessible or distorted rather easily, as new information is constantly coming in. Interestingly, the act of retrieval—recalling something from either memory—is, in itself, an event, and therefore stored in episodic memory. For example, if the clinician encounters a client and retrieves a diagnosis of 'grieving' from semantic memory, the entire situation including the salient features of the grieving diagnosis is stored, at least temporarily, in the episodic memory. The recollection of the situation is likely to change over time as new episodes occur. In contrast to episodic memory, semantic memory probably changes much less often. It is not affected by the act of retrieval, and information in it is more likely to stay there.

The semantic LTM, containing all of the biomedical and nursing knowledge, is comprised of a vast network of associated concepts. There are many theories describing the organization of knowledge in memory; the current evidence is that biomedical knowledge is stored in a *hierarchical* manner, wherein abstract concepts are linked with less abstract examples of that concept. These hierarchically organized concepts with their attendant examples of subconcepts comprise the packets of information retrieved in any diagnostic task.

A hypothetical example of a portion of biomedical knowledge organized hierarchically is depicted in Figure 3–1. Note that the highest level (location) is the most abstract, and subsumes the levels below it. This organization is very important in the diagnostic process. Some studies have shown that diagnostic hypotheses are activated by moving from the more general to the more specific in a top-down fashion, commencing at the lowest possible level (Elstein et al., 1972; Kassirer and Gorry, 1978). For example, based on little data, physicians determine that signs and symptoms are probably related to a cerebellar problem, then progress to identifying the more specific etiological possibilities for the specific disease state, such as degeneration related to alcoholism. Associated with each disease state is information about specific signs and symptoms as well as the alternative treatment regimens.

The packets of information held in LTM may be likened to books stored in a library. They are catalogued by author and title as well as by subject and are placed on shelves by an indexing system (*e.g.*, the Dewey Decimal System). The greater the degree of cross-indexing, for example, the more relevant the subjects under which the book is catalogued, the easier it is for the user to retrieve the needed book.

Such cross-indexing in the nursing knowledge file is exemplified in Figure 3–2. The nurse who is doing a comprehensive assessment using the daily-living model will retrieve the category of ADL and assess the client in the areas of hygiene, nutrition, and so on. Each of these areas will also have a packet of information. If the nurse notes excess body weight, she can retrieve from LTM a packet of information telling her the diagnostic possibilities for excess body weight. She can then retrieve additional files for each of the diagnostic possibilities that would indicate other cues present as well as relevant treatment regimes. Note also that the particular file is cross-indexed with relevant biomedical knowledge.

The signs and symptoms associated with each of the lower levels in the hierarchy are also true of, and associated with, the higher level categories. The coalescing of properties into several categories is essential to success in any diagnostic task. The diagnostician must be able to retrieve the category or categories that are associated with the cues at the appropriate level of abstraction. If she retrieves only one

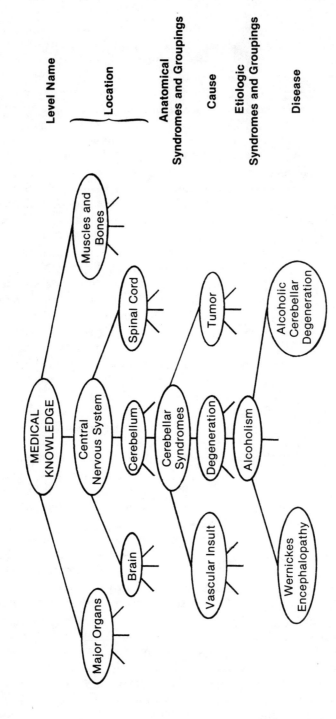

FIG. 3–1. Hypothetical example of medical knowledge organized hierarchically (Wortman, 1972, p. 317).

NURSING KNOWLEDGE FILE

ADL

Hygiene
Nutrition
Cognition
Mobility
See Also Resources, Internal & External
    Health Status, Developmental Tasks

EXCESS BODY WEIGHT

: NUTRITION: ADL ι
See Also, Health Status: Pathology: Endocrine
    Health Status: Developmental Task
    Resources: Knowledge
    Resources: Desire
    Resources: Courage

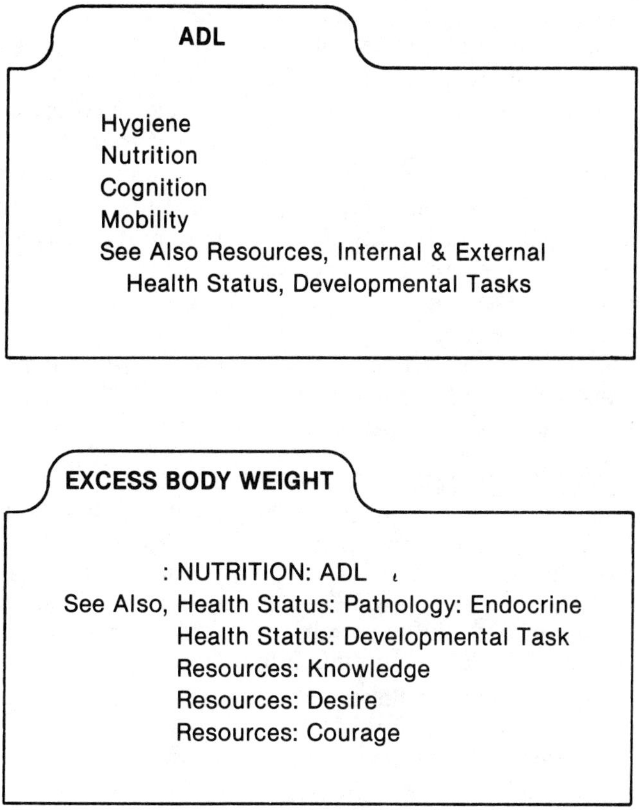

FIG.3–2.   *An example of cross-indexing in the nursing knowledge file.*

category (or one at too specific a level), the correct diagnosis may never be entertained or derived. For example, if the nurse, when encountering an overweight client, retrieves only the packet of information about lack of knowledge, she may fail to gather information about all of the other possible etiologies. She has entered the search field at much too specific a level of abstraction for the presenting cue of excess body weight.

Novices do not have the advantage of this complex, hierarchically organized storehouse of knowledge. Instead, they may hold isolated bits of information but lack the cross-indexing and multiple categorization scheme characteristic of the experts. The formation of a category system can be better understood by examining how the concept of immobility is learned. Students may have learned in basic anatomy, physiology, and pathophysiology that stress on the long bones is necessary for proper calcium metabolism. In another unit, they may have learned that skeletal muscle contraction assists venous return. In basic neuropsychology, they might have learned that a variety of sensory input—through the senses, as well as proprioceptal innervation—is necessary to maintain normal cognitive functioning. These are all bits of information relevant to clinical practice; however, their relevance is apparent only when they are reorganized under the concept of immobility. The clinician can then recognize the need to assess the client for evidence of the untoward sequelae to immobility—renal calculi, venous thrombosis, or impaired cognition due to sensory alteration.

This complex hierarchical network of knowledge with categories, subcategories, and linkages between them serves several important functions for the expert diagnostician:

It saves room in long-term memory.

Retrieval of a category of information with its attendant
subcategories and properties occupies little space in
short-term memory. It further allows the diagnostician
to categorize incoming information from the client,
reducing the cognitive strain that would normally be
produced by large amounts of data.

The organization permits rapid learning. Since a complex
filing system is already established, new information is
more easily categorized and filed for retrieval.

The organization allows for efficient storage of
information from episodic memory. A particular
patient situation stored in episodic memory may be
coded and classified in several categories of diagnostic
information held in semantic memory; this experience
may be used more accurately as a reference point for
later diagnostic tasks than if stored only in episodic
memory.

PROBABILITIES, MEMORY, AND DIAGNOSIS

There is a vast amount of knowledge stored by the clinical expert. The way in which this knowledge is organized, coded and retrieved influences virtually every step of the clinical decision-making process. Its organization and efficient retrieval allows the clinician to reduce the complexity of the task environment, conserving information-processing resources in short-term memory by:

- □ Structuring the clinicians's initial observations and recognition of relevant cues, allowing him/her to ignore irrelevant cues;
- □ Clustering cues into related "chunks,"
- □ Determining which diagnostic hypotheses will be activated,
- □ Forming the substance of the diagnostic hypotheses,
- □ Guiding the search for additional clinical data and for information about risk factors,
- □ Identifying and selecting from alternative courses of treatment.

Several studies on diagnostic reasoning have found that diagnostic categories or hypotheses seemingly "pop into" the clinician's mind almost before the interview with the client begins. Because the nature of the categories retrieved (*e.g.*, level of abstraction, and comprehensiveness of possibilities, associated subcategories, and cues) is related to thoroughness and efficiency of data gathering as well as diagnostic accuracy, it is important to understand what triggers the categories.

It is clear from our preceding discussion that the organization of LTM is a critical determinant in what category is actuated. A cue received from the client must have strong linkages to subcategories stored in LTM; the subcategories must in turn be associated with several larger categories. The category(ies) retrieved by the perfect diagnostician will be at the appropriate level of abstraction *to subsume all subcategories associated with the cue.* For example, the cue *excessive body weight* should activate the categories: nutrition (subsumed under ADL), endocrine pathology (subsumed under health status), and knowledge, desire and courage (subsumed under internal resources).

But our understanding of the organization of LTM is not sufficient to explain how the diagnostic categories are activated. How would the diagnostician decide, in the preceding example, that the category of resources is more likely an explanation for excessive body weight than endocrine pathology? This is where the notion of probabilities enters.

In our earlier discussion, it was noted that diagnostic tasks are characterized by uncertain, probabilistic relationships between cues and diagnoses—for example, that excessive body weight is *probably* associated with lack of desire or courage to stick with a weight reduction diet and *less likely* to be associated with endocrine pathology. The clinician's knowledge of these probabilistic relationships *may* derive from actuarial or incidence data—that in the population at large, the most common cause of obesity is overeating and an infrequent cause is endocrine pathology. Ideally, the expert clinician would use such data as a heuristic both to assist in retrieval of diagnostic categories and, once retrieved, to rank order the likelihood of the competing diagnoses. In other words, the category that would first pop into the clinician's mind would be the most likely, *and* the assessment of its being most likely would be based on real data.

In practice, however, several biases influence the assignment of probabilities and therefore may influence which diagnostic categories are considered. These biases derive largely from our memory of experiences stored in episodic memory. We use our experiences with events to make probability statements about the likelihood of events occurring in the future. For example, a nursing student, about to provide care to a 40-year-old multipara who just gave birth to an unplanned child, might recall: "I remember what it was like for my mother when my brother was born." Based on her experience, she may assign a high probability to coping problems, higher than would be expected if based solely on true incidence rates had they been available.

A series of studies conducted by Kahneman and Tversky (Kahneman and Tversky, 1972; Tversky and Kahneman, 1973, 1974, 1981) revealed biases which may be introduced to the assessment of probabilities. Extending their ideas, it is speculated that three main biases, based in our experience, may influence both the assessment of likelihood of diagnoses and the ease with which diagnostic categories are retrieved.

The first bias is *frequency* of occurrence in our own experience. If we frequently observe that patients in the critical-care unit experience sensory/perceptual alterations, we may conclude that this is always the case. The probability assignment would then be 100%. Our assessment of probability may match objective data but often the sample from which we draw our assessments may be both small and biased. We may observe only three patients in the critical care unit and note that all three experienced some degree of sensory alteration. If we increase the sample of our observations to 10 patients, we might find that the probability of this problem is much less than 100% and we might find some group of patients who are higher risk than others. Furthermore, our sample may be biased by inclusion of only those who indeed are at high risk—the elderly with limitations in hearing and eyesight or those with a high degree of sleep deprivation. If the sample were truly representative of all patients in critical care, our estimate of frequency might be much less.

The assessment of *frequency* influences the diagnostic process by altering the diagnostic possibilities considered. If a critically ill patient displays signs and symptoms of sensory/perceptual alteration *and* if we have assessed the frequency of this problem as 100%, it may be the only diagnosis considered. If, instead, we have assessed the frequency as 20%, we may not activate this diagnostic category at all, or we may be open to considering competing explanations.

A second bias to probability estimates, and to retrieval of diagnostic hypotheses, is *recency of experience*. In making probability estimates, we tend to oversample more recent experiences and to undersample or ignore less recent experiences. If we have just cared for a patient with a sensory/perceptual alteration, we may place a higher probability of this problem's occurrence on the next patient we care for.

This bias was demonstrated in a study of diagnostic processes used by nursing students (Tanner, 1977). The students were presented with a patient situation in which the most likely diagnosis was a sensory alteration. The patient was a 68-year-old diabetic woman who had been hospitalized in the coronary care unit for 5 days. She had had a cataract removal several years before and also had impaired hearing. This situation portrayed the patient experiencing disorientation to time and place and distortion of events surrounding her. Students who had just studied diabetes were convinced, despite absence of confirming data, that the patient was developing insulin reaction; they considered few competing explanations. Students who had just studied neurological disorders were equally convinced that these were early signs of increased intracranial pressure. The recency of the topic under study greatly influenced the probability estimates and the activation of relevant diagnostic categories.

A third bias is introduced by the *profoundness of memory*. We tend to oversample events that are dramatic to us. A group of investigators recently interviewed practicing nurses asking them to describe a patient situation which was typical of the kind of judgments nurses make. We expected to hear reports of decisions about administration of pain medications or recommendations for home health care. Instead, many of the reports were of unusual situations, frequently dramatic rather than typical. Such recollection may bias the probability assigned to diagnoses and the ease with which we retrieve diagnostic hypotheses.

These three biases can profoundly influence the outcome of the diagnostic process. They are no doubt present in diagnosis largely because of the limited processing capacity of STM. The diagnostician must find a means to reduce the range of alternative diagnoses considered at any one time. This is accomplished through the informal assignment of probabilities to competing diagnoses. Objective data regarding frequency of given diagnoses are often not available; and if they are available, the complexity of juggling probabilities and revising them in light of new data may far exceed the processing resources of STM.

The use of experience as a means to retrieve and modify diagnostic hypotheses is not an inherently faulty strategy. Rather, it may be viewed as a resource that can result in effective and efficient diagnostic reasoning *if* one recognizes the potential bias introduced. What distinguishes the novice diagnostician from the expert may be the extent to which the semantic LTM is developed and the extent to which experiences in episodic memory influence the use of knowledge in diagnosis.

THE NOVICE AND THE EXPERT

We have discussed two main factors that influence the diagnostic process—the nature of diagnostic tasks and the characteristics of the diagnostician. It is likely that the novice and the expert differ both in their perception of diagnostic task characteristics and in the extent to which the knowledge store in LTM is developed. These differences, in turn, are likely to influence the strategies adopted for diagnostic problem-solving. We have implied throughout our discussion ways in which novices and experts may differ with respect to these major influencing factors. In this section, we will explicitly *speculate* on the nature of these differences. A comparison of the novice and expert diagnostician is summarized in Table 3–1.

The first difference lies in the perception of the probabilistic nature of diagnostic task. *Novice* diagnosticians may assume that there is a perfect relationship between the presence of a cue and a given diagnosis. Stated another way, if a cue is present, there is a 100% chance of a certain diagnosis. The failure to recognize the prob-

Table 3–1

**Factors Influencing the Diagnostic Process:
Comparison of the Novice and Expert**

Factor	*Novice*	*Expert*
Perception of Task	1. May not recognize probabilistic relationship between cues and diagnosis	1. Recognizes fallibility of cues as indicators of diagnosis

Table 3–1   (*continued*)

Factor	*Novice*	*Expert*
	2. Observations and inferences are treated equally	2. Seeks multiple, dependable, and redundant cues to make inferences
	3. Once recognizes probabilistic relationship, may seek only highly dependable data	3. Weighs risk to patient before seeking more dependable data
	4. Little tolerance for uncertainty in diagnosis	4. High tolerance for uncertainty
Use of Experience	1. Little range and depth of experience	1. Wide range and more depth of experience
	2. Limited experience is used to assign probabilities	2. Experiential sample is more likely to be adequate so chance for bias is reduced
Long-term Memory	1. Categories and subcategories are formed but are limited in number and capacity	1. Hierarchical organization of categories and subcategories
	2. Linkages between categories are few	2. Complex network of linkages between categories
	3. Single cues associated with diagnostic categories	3. Multiple cues and cue patterns cross-referenced to multiple diagnostic categories
	4. Retrieval may be in form of "memorized lists" triggered by a category label	4. Retrieval demonstrates complex network, triggered by category label, subcategory cue, or cue pattern (including risk factors as well as manifestations of problem)

abilistic relationship results in confusing a fact with an inference. Consider the example presented earlier in the chapter in which the novice assumed a perfect relationship between living in a mobile home with poor financial status. The inference of poor financial status was taken as fact and led to a whole series of potentially inaccurate conclusions. The expert, on the other hand, presumably recognizes this probabilistic relationship and, as a result, will seek more dependable cues, and will look for redundant information between cues.

In the *middle*, between the novice and the expert, is the clinician who has recognized the probabilisitic relationship and seeks to accumulate data that will maximally reduce the uncertainty, even though it may not be in the best interest of the client. It has been found, for example, that medical students tend to order sophisticated, costly, and high-risk diagnostic tests (which are dependable indicators of a diagnosis) when, in fact, a more thorough history or a low-risk treatment plan would sufficiently reduce the uncertainty. The *expert* is characterized by her ability to accumulate less dependable data in order to reduce the risk to the client and to tolerate greater uncertainty in the diagnosis.

A second difference between the novice and the expert is the range of experience available to modify probability estimates. The novice has limited experience from which to sample and therefore has greater chance of introducing bias into retrieving diagnostic hypotheses. The expert, equipped with a wide range of experiences, has the advantage of a larger sample size and less of a chance for bias in sampling.

The third and most obvious difference between the novice and expert diagnostician is the extent to which the knowledge base in LTM is developed. The novice begins to form categories and subcategories but they are limited in number and complexity. There may be single cues associated with diagnostic categories. The expert, on the other hand, has a complex network of categories and subcategories. There are multiple cross-references between concepts. Rather than single cues being associated with diagnostic categories, patterns of cues with explicit conditional probabilities are the rule. The expert has also formed special categories which may have derived from experience, such as conditions needing immediate attention.

Because experts hold a complex network of knowledge, they are able to access diagnostic categories efficiently either by single cues or patterns of cues, or by association with other diagnostic categories. For example, with the cues of immobility and frail elderly status, the expert diagnostician can retrieve multiple diagnostic categories related to immobility risk factors such as decubiti, renal calculi, and thrombophlebitis. The beginner may not trigger these risk categories by the presence of the cue *immobility*. But, if given the category label, decubitis ulcer, the novice can list its signs and symptoms and indicate·that the risk is greater with the immobilized, elderly and frail patient. In other words, the retrieval characteristic of the novice may be in the form of *memorized lists*, triggered by a category label.

SUMMARY

The novice and expert differ in the development of their knowledge network and in their perception of the diagnostic task. Both the novice and expert are constrained by the limitations imposed by short-term memory. Because of these limits, both adopt short-cut strategies to deal with the tremendous complexity of diagnosis. That these differences exist between the novice and expert should not be a discouragement for the beginner. Rather, this understanding can be used as a means to develop effective strategies for diagnostic reasoning, which optimizes the use of available knowledge and reduces the untoward consequences of task complexity.

BIBLIOGRAPHY

Elstein AS, Shulman LS and Sprafka SA: Medical Problem-Solving: An Analysis of Clinical Reasoning. Cambridge, Mass.: Harvard University Press, 1978

Hammond KR: Clinical inference in nursing: II. A psychologist's viewpoint. Nursing Research, 15, 27–38, Winter 1966

Kahneman D and Tversky A: Subjective probability: A judgment of representativeness. Cognitive Psychology, 3, 430–454, 1972

Kassirer JP and Gorry CA: Clinical problem-solving: a behavioral analysis. Annals of Internal Medicine, 89, 245–255, 1978

Klatzky RL: Human Memory: Structures and Processes. San Francisco. W.H. Freeman and Company, 1975

Miller CA: The magical number seven, plus or minus two: some limits on our capacity for processing information. Psychological Review, 63, 81–97, 1956

Newel A, Simon HA: Human Problem Solving. Englewood Cliffs, NJ, Prentice-Hall, 1972

Simon HA: Information-processing theory of human problem solving. In Estes WK (ed): Handbook of Cognitive Process, Volume 5: Human Information Processing. Hillsdale, NJ, Laonimc Earlbaum Associates, 1978

Tanner CA: The effect of hypothesis generation as an instructional method on the diagnostic processes of senior baccalaureate nursing students. Unpublished doctoral dissertation. University of Colorado, 1977

Tversky A and Kahneman D: Judgment under uncertainty: Heuristics and Biases. Science, *185*, 1124–1131, 1974

Tversky A and Kahneman D: Availability: A heuristic for judging frequency and probability. Cognitive Psychology, 5, 207–232, 1973

Tversky A and Kahneman D: The framing of decisions and the psychology of choice. Science, 211, 453–458, 1981

Wortman PM: Medical diagnosis: an information processing approach. Computers and Biomedical Research, 5, 315–318, 1972

CHAPTER FOUR

Diagnostic Problem-Solving Strategies

Christine A. Tanner

In the previous chapter, we examined major factors that influence the diagnostic process. It was pointed out that despite holding a huge storehouse of information in LTM, the human problem-solver has a limited capacity to actively handle this information from LTM coupled with information from the environment. Factors that influence the complexity of diagnostic tasks were described; the greater the complexity of the diagnostic task, the greater the cognitive burden. The diagnostician must adopt strategies that will reduce this cognitive burden and that will make most efficient use of limited information-processing resources. In this chapter we will examine more closely the cognitive strategies used in diagnosis, compare the novice and expert in these strategies, and explore ways in which the pitfalls of diagnostic strategies might be avoided.

THE STARTING POINT: NARROWING THE SEARCH FIELD

In any encounter with a client, a tremendous amount of information is potentially available to the clinician—risk factors, physical signs, symptoms, laboratory reports, social history, cultural background, and environmental factors. From this vast field of data, the clinician must select and use the most relevant information when making a clinical judgment. Upon entering a "problem-space" of this complexity, the natural human tendency is to try and narrow the search field, reduce its complexity, and, in essence, define it in such a way that the information-processing capacity can handle it. Hence, even prior to the initial encounter with the client, the search field may be narrowed.

Pre-Encounter Influences

There are several pre-encounter influences which shape the search field. One's discipline orientation (for example, biomedical vs. nursing) as well as one's specialty orientation within the discipline will determine to a great extent the cues which the diagnostician attends to and those which he ignores. Nurses who believe that they are to serve primarily as the eyes and ears of the physician have already narrowed their search field to pathophysiological/biomedical data. Nurses using the daily living model have narrowed their search field to daily-living effectiveness.

Very subtle cues, ones which may not even enter our conscious thinking, also narrow the search field. Benner (1981), in her study of development of nursing expertise, interviewed nurses about situations they encountered. One expert nurse describes an emergency situation in the Intensive Care Unit:

> I had worked late and was just about ready to go home, when a nurse said to me, 'Jolene, come here,' her voice had urgency in it, but not Code Blue. (Benner, 1981, p. 33)

The nurse noted that her colleague's voice had urgency in it, but not a Code Blue urgency. She had noticed the absence of the familiar cues of a cardiac arrest. Such subtle cues can profoundly influence our expectations of the situation and reduce the size of the problem space immensely. Benner points out that this ability to attend to such subtle cues prior to seeing the patient is a function of experience. Novices simply lack the experience needed to grasp the significance of such subtle information.

The environment in which data gathering occurs, and the pre-encounter patient data also shape the search field. As a result of the environment and the limited patient data, certain expectations are formulated; a psychological set is established. For example, a nurse working in a prenatal clinic is about to interview a woman who has come in for a routine six-month prenatal check. The nurse, prior to entering the room, has probably already formulated the initial questions based on these expectations, focusing on aspects such as daily living changes and altering family relationships, which would be anticipated with the arrival of the new baby. Knowing the parity and the age of the client may further focus the nurse's expectations. The client's demands of daily living and external resources are likely to be much different if the woman is a 20-year-old primapara than if she is a 40-year-old multipara. The nurse may not expect other non-pregnancy-related health problems to emerge.

The ability to narrow the search field based on these data results from the knowledge stored in long-term memory. The combination of environmental data and client data serves to activate from LTM a large category of information—not at the specific hypothesis level, but at a level which greatly reduces the scope of the information search. Multiple hypotheses may later be activated as more information is acquired.

This ability to narrow the search field should be viewed as both a resource and an impediment to accurate data collection and diagnosis. The expert can employ the heuristic method fairly reliably by entering the search field with the proper category of information in hand, that which is at the appropriate level of abstraction. The expert with this limited amount of data has not yet activated specific hypotheses that would restrict the search field so much that the relevant data would be missed. The expectations generated from the limited data remain broad enough so that the expert diagnostician can more readily modify his or her expectations on the basis of new data.

Beginners do not have the advantages of the extensive knowledge base or experience held by the expert, so one of two procedures may be used by them. They may proceed along the lines of the classical empiricist, systematically collecting data in the prescribed manner used for all patients. Because of the space limitations in the working memory (STM), they would probably have to rely on using memory aids, such as taking notes, examining the data for "abnormal" findings, then matching the data with textbook descriptions. Only then would the search field begin to narrow significantly.

Beginners may, on the other hand, attempt to use their own life experiences to narrow the range of possibilities ("I remember what it was like for my mother when she was 40 and had my baby brother.") This information is retrieved from episodic memory and does not have the advantage of having been filtered through or linked with the scientific knowledge (e.g., normal development tasks, daily living adjustments) stored in semantic long-term memory. The problem with this approach is that the search field is narrowed much too quickly, the category of information retrieved is much too restrictive, and relevant data is likely to be missed. Even if the beginning clinician is able to determine that what he expected is not supported by subsequent data, a set has already been established. Then it is extremely difficult to entertain other possibilities.

The middle-level clinician, with some knowledge stashed neatly away but without the extensive memory network characteristic of the expert, may experience varying degrees of success using this strategy. The number of categories stored in memory increases with growing expertise—with bits of knowledge being recoded and reclassified in several categories of progressively higher levels of abstraction. The category of knowledge used by the middle-level clinician to narrow the search field may not be as broad, or contain as many elements as the category used by the expert. The result is a search field that is initially too narrow and one in which all the problems with psychological set experienced by the beginner may again rear their ugly heads. In some cases this is not a problem because the category of knowledge retrieved may indeed contain all of the information necessary to derive the accurate diagnosis, despite the fact that the clinician entered the search field with a narrower perspective than that of the expert.

Let's look at another earlier-cited example, and explore some pre-encounter influences. An expert nurse and a student hear the following report:

> Mrs. Jamison is a 63-year-old patient who is 14 days post coronary-artery-bypass-graft surgery. She has been stable, ambulating well in the hallway and making plans to go home. She had a history of increasing angina prior to surgery with no documented M.I. She does have a recent history of peptic ulcer disease, mild chronic lung disease, and rheumatoid arthritis.

The student described her thinking:

> She's making plans to go home and she's been stable. The focus of my attention was figuring out how I would help her get ready for her discharge and finding out what she needed to learn before she leaves the hospital.

The nurse described her thinking:

> This lady has multiple medical problems. She's been stable after surgery and the fact that she had no M.I.'s is in her favor. But all of her problems mean that she'll have a lot to deal with when she goes home. I needed to pay attention to how well she was responding to all her problems—find out what "stable" really meant. I needed to get some baseline before I could think about discharge plans.

The two nurses narrowed their search field dramatically. The novice focused on one cue—preparing for discharge—and expected to find a medically stable patient ready to go home. The expert narrowed her search field in a different way; she wanted to assess the woman's responses to her illnesses and ascertain the meaning of "stable." She expected to find a woman with multiple medical problems and a questionable ability to cope with all of them. When the two nurses entered the room, they found Mrs. Jamison complaining of weakness, being unable to do much for herself, and indicating that she had abdominal pain. The novice, assuming that the cues were all related to Mrs. Jamison's pending discharge proceeded to evaluate what the problems were in her home situation. The expert was more open to difficulties arising from the many medical problems and explored further the nature of the abdominal pain and the weakness. Mrs. Jamison was later diagnosed by the physician as having a bleeding gastric ulcer. The expert nurse's willingness to keep open the search field allowed her to make relevant observations and an appropriate referral.

Initial Data: Entry to the Search Field

When the clinician first meets the client, the search field is further narrowed. Novices and experts alike use cues from the client within the first seconds of the encounter to reduce the size of the search field. There are, however, significant differences in how they approach this initial encounter with the client.

The expert will quickly assess the extent to which prior expectations match observations of the client. Because experts have not significantly narrowed the search field based on pre-encountered data, they are open to, and look for, patterns of cues that do not match expectations. Their approach to the initial encounter is characterized by a collaboration with the client on management of data. They view objective data as cues for subjective verification with the client. Hence, our expert in the preceding example shared with the client her perception that the client might be concerned about going home; the client responded that she was eager to be with her family and was mostly worried about the abdominal pain and her feeling of weakness. The process of verification with the client allowed the expert to focus on significant cues.

Probably the most predominant characteristic of experts in the initial encounter phase is their ability to use cues. Experts differ from novices in their capacities to extract maximal information from available cues and to recognize patterns of cues. Let's compare novice and expert nurses in their approaches to the patient with the likely diagnosis of sensory deprivation. The patient was a 68-year-old diabetic woman who had been hospitalized in the coronary-care use for five days following an M.I. She had had cataract removal several years before and also had impaired hearing. When the nurse entered the room she found the patient out of bed, looking through her bedside stand. The patient stated that she was tired of "those wires" keeping her in bed and that she'd provided enough help in "checking out" the equipment.

The expert described her thinking:

Nurse: Everything was there for CCU-itis. What made me sure of it was her behavior. These patients get confused but their confusion is sort of delusional, like this lady's. She thought the wires were to keep her in bed and that she was there to help make sure the equipment was working.

Interviewer: Did you consider anything else?

Nurse: Well, I had a fleeting thought I guess about some medical problems. I'd want to check that out further, just in case, but the pattern is there for sensory dep.

Interviewer: Can you describe any more about the pattern?

Nurse: If I stop and think about it—limited hearing and vision, CCU for five days, zip meaningful input, you know—no family visiting, pretty much in bed the whole time. It could be other things, but it all fits together.

Notice that the expert extracted a great deal of information from the patient's behavior. She also described how the cues coalesced into a pattern, almost at a preconscious level. She held in the back of her mind other possibilities, wishing to avoid premature closure on the most likely diagnosis. She moved with facility from the biomedical domain to the nursing domain.

The novice described her thinking:

Nurse: Well, this lady was real confused. I'd want to know when she had her last insulin.

Interviewer: What would that information tell you?

Nurse: Well, I think she has a problem with her diabetes. I had another patient once who had a real funny reaction to insulin. Nothing changed—vital signs were OK, skin was OK—except she'd act weird. She'd move slowly and kind of stare into space.

Interviewer: And this patient reminds you of the one you took care of before?

Nurse: Yeah, well, sort of. I mean the confusion is a lot alike.

Interviewer: Can you think of anything else?

Nurse: Well, just stuff about her diabetes—if she's eaten, what her Clinitest was. But, um, I suppose maybe something with her heart. If you don't get enough blood to the brain you can get confused. Or maybe she's just denying her heart attack.

The novice, lacking in both the extensive knowledge base and the range of experience, missed the cue pattern noted by the expert and also did not pick up all the subtleties present in the cue configuration. She had closed in quickly on a biomedical problem and really had to grope to come up with other possibilities.

Benner (1981) maintains that the ability to see such cue patterns is entirely a function of experience, and it may be so. Novices, however, are tooled with the capacity for careful analysis, and if cautious in their approach to avoid the effects of set, can still derive the most likely diagnosis.

HYPOTHESIS ACTIVATION

The coalescing of cues during the initial encounter with the client quickly becomes a process of activating hypotheses. In fact, recognition of familiar cue patterns and the generation of diagnostic hypotheses are complementary strategies that can rarely be separated in practice. The early generation of diagnostic hypotheses is characteristic of both novices and experts. It is the one strategy that is uniformly described in study after study of diagnostic problem-solving processes used by physicians and medical students (Barrows and Bennett, 1972; Ekwo, 1977; Elstein, Shulman and Sprafka, 1978; Kasserir and Gorry, 1978; Neurfeld et al, 1981).

Early hypothesis generation is an important strategy: it is likely that this is the primary way in which clinicians adapt their limited information-processing resources to the demands of complex diagnostic tasks. It is argued that an early hypothesis serves as a "chunking" mechanism in short-term memory, greatly increasing its capacity to hold the huge amount of clinical data provided by the client. Hence, it is posited by these investigators that early hypothesis generation is a strategy used by all clinicians, regardless of their level of clinical knowledge and regardless of discipline orientation, as a means to maximally use resources in short-term memory.

This strategy is greatly influenced by the extent to which the knowledge network in LTM is developed. We discussed, at some length in the preceding chapter, the factors that influence hypothesis activation. Single cues or cue patterns will activate hypotheses if they have cross references to relevant diagnostic categories; the number of hypotheses as well as their level of specificity is determined, in large part, by the elaborations with which LTM knowledge stores are categorized, indexed, and cross referenced. We also discussed the biases that influence both hypothesis activation and evaluation, including the availability of instances and recency and profoundness of experiences.

Let us now examine how a novice and expert approach a patient situation in terms of their activation of diagnostic hypothesis.

> *The Situation:* You are a visiting nurse about to see Mr. Mitchell on a routine-home visit. Mr. Mitchell is a 68-year-old widower who has moderately severe chronic-obstructive-pulmonary disease. He has been on disability for approximately one year. He lives in a one bedroom apartment and manages to do his own shopping and cooking. He has friends in the neighborhood with whom he visits frequently, plays cards and goes fishing. He can usually walk one-half block before developing severe dyspnea. He has oxygen at home, which he uses occasionally.
>
> When you arrive, you note the smell of cigarette smoke permeating the air. Mr. Mitchell is more short of breath than usual. He explains that he went to the "breathing clinic" four days ago because of increased dyspnea and they started him on Prednisone. He indicates that he has gained about eight pounds in the last week. He expresses great frustration at not being able to get out and see his friends—he's tired of being housebound.

The experienced nurse's approach:

Interviewer: Could you tell me what your initial thoughts are?

Nurse: Well, a lot of things bother me—weight gain, that he's probably smoking again, his increased shortness of breath and his being upset that he can't get out with his friends anymore. This isn't a real unusual situation—these people get into trouble, go into the hospital, get patched up, go home where they have no resources, and 'boom' end up in trouble again. He's got a physical problem with the weight gain, shortness of breath, decreased activity tolerance, and Prednisone isn't helping. All these things could be related, or maybe not—he could be into cor pulmonale, or developing a pulmonary infection. Oh, another thing, if he's not getting out, I wonder how he's eating. He could be 'upping' his salt intake. That could be a problem. Prednisone also causes fluid retention plus his disease process.

But I'm also gonna want to deal with his smoking; you know, check that out with him to see if he is. And he's pretty upset and lonely so I'd want to explore that more with him. They might all be hooked up together, and maybe not, but I think I want to find out first about his eating—see if we can put together his immobility and his weight gain and breathing problems.

Interviewer: Anything else in your initial thoughts?

Nurse: No, just those three big things—his frustration at not being able to get out, the physical problem, and smoking—which could all be linked up together or all separate.

The expert's approach is characterized by the coalescing of cues into patterns. She is attempting first to see if the majority of the cues can be explained by a limited number of hypotheses. She combined the information about Prednisone and the possibility of an increased salt intake into a hypothesis of fluid retention leading to weight gain and increased shortness of breath. The shortness of breath, in turn, might explain his inability to get out with friends. At the same time, she mentioned more specific hypotheses in the biomedical domain—cor pulmonale and pulmonary infection, and she's holding the possibility that he's still smoking for further exploration. In this case, the strategy was to find the hypothesis that explained most of the cues, generating competing explanations and noting cues in need of further examination. The expert is able to move with facility from abstract hypotheses to very specific ones.

Now let's examine the novice nurse's approach to the same situation:

Interviewer: Could you tell me what your initial thoughts are?

Nurse: I think he's uh . . . for some reason gotten to the point where he's having a whole lot of trouble coping with his life the way it is now. And it could be that he's approaching some kind of pivotal point in his life where he's going to need . . . uh . . . I wouldn't say hospitalization or institutionalization, but some kind of structured help to come in. More than a home visit once a week-type of thing. Um, that's my initial impression of the situation. Ah . . . he's got a problem with his steroid and I think I want to find out what other medication he's taking. Start out with the physical picture.

Interviewer: You say he has problems coping. Could you describe that a bit more for me?

Nurse: Well, he said he couldn't get out to see his buddies anymore. He might do better if he were living in a place where friends were nearer.

Interviewer: And you mentioned problems with Prednisone.

Nurse: Yes, he's gained eight pounds and Prednisone causes weight gain. Don't know if, uh, it can cause eight pounds to go on, but, uhm, it could.

Interviewer: Anything else that you are thinking about now?

Nurse: No, I just need to know more about the physical picture—what meds he's on.

The novice's approach is different than that of the expert. She too activated hypotheses—one that was very general, describing "difficulty coping with his life the way it is now," and one that linked the weight gain to Prednisone. It appears that the novice has difficulty in coalescing the cues into a common pattern. She appears to be dealing with only two cues in the biomedical domain (weight-gain and Prednisone). Because she's considering changing his home care, one might infer that she does not link, at least at this point, his social isolation with an acute biomedical problem, as the expert was hypothesizing. She seemed to ignore (or not actively consider) the multiple remaining cues presented: his changes in nutrition, his increased shortness of breath, and his smoking.

Several explanations may account for this difference. The two nurses may differ only in what they describe their thinking to be, not in the actual strategies themselves. Only further analysis of data with several individuals will rule out or confirm this explanation. It is likely that the novice does not have the complex network of information in LTM, so it would be difficult to link all the presenting cues with fluid retention. Lacking the knowledge network in LTM, and hence, the capacity to "chunk" cues, it's also possible that the novice had difficulty retaining all the bits of information in STM. Hence she did not attend to his smoking, shortness of breath, and nutritional changes.

In sum, then, novices seem to differ from experts in the early hypothesis-activation stage along three dimensions:

☐ Experts use cue patterns as sources for hypothesis while novices rely more heavily on single cues.

☐ Experts seek hypotheses at a level of abstraction necessary to explain as many cues as possible, while novices tend to have either very general or very specific hypotheses.

☐ Experts hold in reserve for later exploration those cues that can not be explained with existing hypotheses, while novices may not attend to the cues. Studies of medical students suggest that they differ from their physician counterparts in the number of cues explained by hypotheses and the level of abstraction (Elstein et al, 1978; Neufeld et al, 1981).

The preceding portrayal is not intended to be disheartening for the novice, but rather reflects differences one might expect due to differences in knowledge and level of experience. Some very effective strategies can be adopted during the data gathering to assist the novice in avoiding premature closure and in deriving the most likely diagnosis.

GUIDED SEARCH

Having initially activated diagnostic hypotheses, a general strategy adopted by both novice and expert clinicians is to go about gathering data in order to systematically test the hypotheses (Elstein et al, 1978; Kassirer and Gorry, 1978; Barrows and Bennett, 1972; Gordon, 1980; Neufield et al, 1981). In other words, the clinician actively considers one or more hypotheses and gathers data that will assist in either confirming or ruling out the hypothesis. Kassirer and Gorry (1978) described four specific strategies used by expert physicians.

□ A *confirmation* strategy, in which the clinician seeks data that would prove a hypothesis by matching the characteristics of the clinical state under consideration.

□ An *elimination* strategy uses questions about findings associated so often with a given disease that their absence weighs heavily against the hypothesized disease.

□ A *discrimination* strategy used to distinguish one hypothesis from another.

□ An *exploration* strategy used to refine a hypothesis by making it more specific and to check for related or unrelated disorders or complications.

Obviously, such facility with questioning requires a great deal of knowledge about the hypothesized condition. And it seems that even experts get stumped. The experts frequently shift a questioning approach from hypothesis-testing to asking questions that are part of a routine inquiry (Barrows & Bennett, 1972). They do this when the hypothesis-testing is no longer productive, thereby continuing to ask questions until a positive finding is elicited, then returning to hypothesis-testing. At times, they may wish to ponder the problem without disrupting the interview. Routine questioning is also an important part of the expert's repertoire to avoid premature closure on an obvious conclusion.

Let's examine our expert nurse's information-seeking strategies from the previous example. We left her at the point where she was planning to explore fluid retention, related to increased sodium intake, and Prednisone.

Nurse: I imagine it's been difficult for you to prepare meals for yourself. How have you managed?

Patient: There's a restaurant across the street so I've been eating once or twice a day over there. I'm getting pretty tired of the menu.

Nurse: What sorts of things are on the menu?

Patient: The usual fast-food fare—hamburgers, chicken, cole slaw, fries. I ask them not to salt the fries.

Nurse: So you've been trying to hold back on the salt.
Could you tell me what you eat on a typical day?

Patient: For lunch, a hamburger or tuna sandwich. For
dinner, fried chicken or shrimp and cole slaw.
Sometimes fries.

Nurse: Mr. Mitchell, I'm thinking that perhaps the reason
you've put on so much weight and have trouble
breathing is from fluid retention. The foods you
describe in your diet have a lot of salt and that
could cause you to hold water. It sounds like your
big worry now is being able to get out with your
friends.

Patient: Yeah, it is. I really am sick of feeling this way.

Nurse: Well, I hope that if we can find some of the reasons
for your increased shortness of breath, we'll be able
to help you return to your usual activities. How
long have you been eating at the restaurant?

Patient: I guess about a week, maybe a little less.

The nurse proceeded to check Mr. Mitchell's ankles for swelling,
noting 1^+ edema, and listened to his lungs, finding scattered ronchi
and rales. She describes her thinking as follows:

> Well, it was beginning to sound more and more like
> a problem with fluid retention. I still didn't know what
> took him to the pulmonary clinic last week, but I'd check
> that out later. Now I was beginning to wonder whether
> his diet change was only a lack of external resources or
> whether he didn't know about the sodium amount in the
> foods he was eating, or whether he'd gotten so down in
> the dumps that he'd given up trying to stick with the
> medical regimen. And his smoking clicked in here.

The nurse was using a confirmation strategy, seeking data about
the main hypothesis of fluid retention. She also recognized that she
needed to attend to Mr. Mitchell's primary concern and to share her
observations with him. As she obtained information, she began to
refine her hypothesis, seeking an explanation for the diet change.
This *"stringing together of concepts"* (edema, shortness of breath,
weight gain, fluid retention, increased sodium intake, lack of knowledge about diet, lack of ability to prepare diet, lack of desire to main-

tain) is not an unusual strategy employed by experts during the information-gathering phase (Kassirer and Gorry, 1978).

Now let's examine the questioning approach used by the novice. (In this situation, the nurse is asking an examiner for the information she would obtain from the patient.)

Nurse: First I would want to know what medications he was on.

Examiner: Digoxin .25 mg qd, HCTZ 50 mg bid, KCL 20 mEq bid, Prednisone 40 mg qd, Theodor 300 mg qid.

Nurse: HCTZ could be for blood pressure. What's his blood pressure?

Examiner: 140/90.

Nurse: Hmm, that might be what it's for, but it could be for fluid problems. And Prednisone could cause fluid retention. He shouldn't have a problem with fluid if he's on HCTZ. His smoking history, I wondered if he's smoking.

Examiner: He smokes about ½ pack per day. He has a 30-year history of 2 packs a day, and in the last 6 months cut back to half a pack a day.

Nurse: Is there any indication that he's increased his smoking in the last, you know, couple of weeks or months?

Examiner: No, he's trying to quit.

Nurse: I think his physical problems, they seem to be stemming from his respiratory problems. Ahm, his hypertension is borderline. What happened to him in the breathing clinic? Uh, what did they find?

The nurse describes her thinking at this point:

I'm trying to figure out his breathing problems. That seems to be the main problem. I guess I'm stumped and I thought I'd see if there are any clues in, you know, his record from the clinic visit.

The novice asked a few hypothesis-testing questions and she related her findings of HCTZ to her hypothesis about fluid retention.

The other strategy she used might be labeled a data-driven search (rather than hypothesis-driven). She asked clarifying questions about each cue, and probably clustered the subsequent data she obtained around each cue as a means to conserve space in STM. The approach to cue characterization may be useful and prevent premature closure on an inaccurate hypothesis. When stumped, she returned to more general questions, searching for information that would help her make some meaning about the data she already obtained.

It's interesting to note that much later in the testing, this nurse returned to the question of smoking. She also wondered out loud if the patient was taking his HCTZ and stumbled on the possibility that he wasn't sticking to the medical regimen. Having retrieved the category of noncompliance, she asked further questions about his diet. Her final diagnosis was lack of knowledge about dietary regimen.

A pattern frequently used by experts and occasionally by novices is resorting to routine general questions. A nurse who would ask the patient general questions about daily-living patterns would eventually find the needed information to make the accurate diagnosis. In fact, the switch to routine questions adopted by experts may be a strategy useful in avoiding premature closure.

In summary, novices may be contrasted with experts in their guided search strategies in the following dimensions:

- Both use hypothesis-testing strategies, although the experts tend to be more complete in their initial set of hypotheses and more thorough in their testing of hypotheses.

- Both use a general routine questioning strategy. Like novices, experts evoke its use when stumped. In addition, experts use it as a means to avoid premature closure.

- Both use cue characterization, but much of the novice's information-seeking is characterized by questions to explore cues (data driven). The expert uses the strategy to test or refine hypotheses.

- Experts are able to use all strategies with great facility. They can readily shift the focus of the search in light of new information and new priorities. Novices, on the other hand, have difficulty in shifting their strategies. They may quickly abandon a focus of the search in light of new data, but unlike experts, may fail to return to the original focus.

HYPOTHESIS EVALUATION

Evaluation of diagnostic hypotheses is an integral component of the stage of information-seeking. The process of evaluation is one of continuously weighing the probability of each active hypothesis with each new piece of information obtained from the client. Hence, it requires the juggling of probabilities: with this cue, the probability of Hypothesis 1 increases and the probability of Hypothesis 2 decreases. Therefore, the ability to effectively evaluate hypotheses is related to one's understanding of the relationship between each cue and each hypothesis. It is also related to one's ability to identify and seek the cue or cues that lead to the greatest revision of the probability of a hypothesis.

One might view hypothesis evaluation as establishing a certain threshold. If the probability of a hypothesis exceeds the threshold, then the diagnosis is accepted. If the probability fails to exceed the threshold because of disconfirming data, then it is rejected. Obviously diagnosticians do not assign real numbers to the probability statements, but there probably exists informal rank-ordering of hypotheses, such as: it is more likely to be Hypothesis 1 than Hypothesis 2.

The other factor profoundly influencing hypothesis evaluation is the probability that the hypothesis holds before any data is accumulated. In our discussion in the preceding chapter, it was noted that three biases influence the retrieval and probability estimates of the initial hypotheses: availability of instances, recency, and profoundness. Let us say, for example, that a critical-care nurse has frequently encountered many patients with sensory deprivation, all of whom experienced the condition recently. As a result, she assigned a 90% probability to sensory deprivation as the hypothesis explaining her current patient's signs and symptoms. It may take a great deal more disconfirming data to reject this hypothesis than if it had been assigned the probability of 40%. If a single diagnostic hypothesis is the only one retrieved, then it may hold an inappropriately high probability and will be more difficult to reject.

It is likely that expert and novice performances will differ on hypothesis evaluation, again primarily because of differences in knowledge-base and levels of experience. Experts seek and use data that have the greatest probability of confirming the diagnosis, ruling out the diagnosis, or differentiating between two competing hypotheses (Kassirer and Gorry, 1978). Hence, they tend to be more efficient in their data-gathering and hypothesis evaluation. They are able to use confirming and disconfirming data equally well and cautiously avoid jumping to conclusions on the basis of a single cue.

The novices, on the other hand, may lack the knowledge necessary to select the most useful cues for evaluating hypotheses. As a result, they tend to gather more data before accepting a hypothesis. Novices also appear to underestimate the information value of disconfirming information and they may overestimate the value of confirming information (Tanner, 1977; Matthews and Gaul, 1979). This characteristic is especially true when the novice diagnostician has only one active hypothesis. It may result from a psychological set toward the favored (or only) hypothesis leading to an overzealous acceptance of data that support the favorite hypothesis and a virtual bypass of data that do not.

Table 4–1

Diagnostic Strategies:
The Novice and the Expert

Phase of Diagnostic Process	Novice	Expert
Narrowing the Search Field	1. Stereotypes on basis of pre-encounter information	1. Uses pre-encounter data to expedite early directed data search. Validates with data in presenting situation
	2. Uses general systematic search; relies on memory of past experiences to narrow search field	2. Begins with general systematic search to avoid premature narrowing
	3. Looks for data that confirm pre-encounter influence	3. Looks for data which differ from pre-encounter expectations
	4. May miss patterns in cues	4. Recognizes patterns in cues
	5. Does not realize full information value from cues to narrow search field	5. Extracts maximal information from cues to narrow search field
Hypothesis Activation	1. Uses single cues to trigger hypotheses	1. Uses cue patterns/ clusters as triggers for hypotheses

Table 4–1   (*continued*)

Phase of Diagnostic Process	Novice	Expert
	2. Hypotheses are very global or very specific; level of specificity may not fit data	2. Seeks hypotheses at level of abstraction necessary to explain as much of the data as possible
	3. May ignore or forget cues that do not fit hypotheses	3. Holds in reserve for later exploration cues that cannot be "chunked" into the hypotheses activated
Information-seeking	1. Uses hypothesis testing to a limited degree	1. Uses hypothesis testing efficiently and more thoroughly than novice
	2. Usually uses routine general questioning strategy when stumped	2. Uses routine general questioning strategy when stumped and as a means to avoid premature closure
	3. Uses cue characterization or data-driven searches as primary approach	3. Uses cue characterization as a means to test or refine hypotheses
	4. Has difficulty shifting focus of search and strategy	4. Can shift focus and strategy with great facility
	5. May be uncomfortable validating with client	5. Validates with client
Hypothesis Evaluation	1. Uses recency of experience and availability to assess likelihood of hypothesis	1. Uses more reliable sample (wide range of experience) to assess likelihood
	2. Nonselective in data obtained	2. Uses data with greatest information value

Table 4–1   (*continued*)

Phase of Diagnostic Process	Novice	Expert
	3. Tends to gather either too much or too little data depending on initial probability	3. Efficient in data gathering and hypothesis evaluation
	4. Underestimates value of disconfirming data and overestimates value of confirming data	4. Information value less influenced by confirming/disconfirming nature
	5. Tendency toward premature closure on favored hypothesis	5. Recognizes the importance of avoiding premature closure

SUMMARY

In this chapter, we have considered the strategies employed by both novices and experts in the diagnostic process. The comparison between the two groups is summarized in Table 4–1. The experts are those who efficiently narrow the search field based on patterns of cues and extract maximal information from cues. The cue patterns serve as bases for early hypothesis, generated within seconds to minutes of the initial encounter with the client. They seek hypotheses that explain as many of the cues as possible, holding in reserve for later exploration those that remain unexplained. Their search strategies are generally hypothesis-driven and quite efficient, but they move with facility to other strategies when needed. They readily seek validation with the client, having adopted the collaborative approach to data management. Experts gather data with the greatest information value, evaluating each active hypothesis with each new cue. They adopt strategies that prevent premature closure.

Just as there are no diagnosticians who match this description completely, there are also no diagnosticians who commit all the errors attributed to the novice. Expert diagnosticians are subject to the commitment of human errors and novices are frequently able to employ appropriate strategies for diagnosis. The single greatest variable influencing diagnoses is the extent to which the knowledge network is developed in LTM. Given a sometimes-limited knowledge-base, novices can perform surprisingly well in many situations. Indeed, the strategies they seem to adopt naturally assist them in many ways.

Some Tips For Improving Diagnosis

If you found yourself identifying more closely with the novice than the expert, take heart. There are some ways in which you can improve your diagnostic-reasoning skills. At the core of the following suggestions is a single yet very important research finding: the best predictor of diagnostic accuracy is thoroughness of data collection—not the elegance of narrowing the search field, not the brilliance of the hypotheses, not the efficiency of cue acquisition.

- □ Remember that cues are less-than-perfect indicators of the diagnosis, not the same as the diagnosis.
- □ Be cautious when separating observations from inferences. It is easy for us to leap from a fact to a conclusion without ever knowing we did it.
- □ When you observe a sign or symptom, don't settle for the first explanation that comes to mind. Always look for competing diagnoses.
- □ Try to consider two to three diagnoses at one time. When you get additional information, consider each diagnosis in light of the new information. Check to be sure that competing diagnoses have been ruled out, or can wait until you've tried some competing interventions.
- □ Follow up on each cue. Explore its characteristics, watching carefully for the influence of biases or your favored hypothesis on the kind of questions you ask.
- □ Validate both your observations and your inferences with your client.
- □ As you narrow the range of diagnostic possibilities, go back and evaluate what data led you to favor one diagnosis and begin to rule out others.

> Are the data reliable and dependable indicators of your diagnosis?
>
> Was your diagnosis influenced by a recent experience or dramatic event?

Are the diagnostic possibilities reminiscent of another client situation? And if so, is the client you recall representative of a larger group of clients?

□ Be cautious of premature closure. Remember the information we obtain from a client and the observations we make are determined largely by what we think the diagnostic possibilities are. Don't abandon routine general questioning too quickly. While focused data collection is efficient, failure to uncover problems in daily living can come from a premature narrowing of the search field.

□ Be tentative in your diagnosis. There is seldom a time when all uncertainty can be removed. The final diagnosis is at best a conjecture. The process of collaborative diagnosis with the client may in itself be therapeutic. It may assist the client to sufficiently mobilize resources such that no further intervention is needed.

□ Be confident in your reasoning skills and your ability to draw accurate inferences. As a nurse, you have finely-tuned observation skills and a vast storehouse of knowledge. Belief in your own ability coupled with an open, inquisitive mind go a long way toward effective problem-solving.

BIBLIOGRAPHY

Barrows HS and Bennet K: The diagnostic problem-solving task of the neurologist. *Archives of Neurology 62:* 273–277, 1972

Benner P, Colavecchio R, Field K and Gordon D: From Novice to Expert: A Community View of Preparing and Rewarding Excellence in Clinical Nursing Practice. *U of Calif, San Francisco:* AMICAE Project, 1981

Ekwo EE: An analysis of the problem-solving process of third year medical students. In Proceedings of the 16th Annual Conference on Research in Medical Education. Washington, D.C. Association of American Medical Colleges, 1977

Elstein AS, Shulman LS and Sprafka SA: Medical Problem-Solving: An Analysis of Clinical Reasoning. Cambridge, Mass.: Harvard University Press, 1978

Gordon M: Predictive strategies in diagnostic tasks. *Nursing Research 29:* 39–45, 1980

Kassirer JP and Gorry CA: Clinical problem-solving: a behavioral analysis. Annals of Internal Medicine *89:* 245–255, 1978

Matthews CA and Gaul AL: Nursing diagnosis from the perspective of concept attainment. Advances in Nursing Science 1: 17–26, 1979

Neufeld VR, Norman GR, Feightner JW and Barrow HS: Clinical problem-solving by medical students: a cross sectional and longitudinal analysis. Medical Education 15: 315–322, 1981

Tanner CA: The effect of hypothesis generation as an instructional method on the diagnostic processes of senior baccalaureate nursing students. Unpublished doctoral dissertation. University of Colorado, 1977

SECTION THREE

Diagnostic Reasoning in Clinical Practice
Pamela H. Mitchell

Overview

Section Three demonstrates the diagnostic reasoning process as it is used by nurses working in a variety of clinical settings. These chapters were written by practicing specialists, the majority of whom are faculty members of a school of nursing. The contributors met over a considerable period of time attempting to clarify and make explicit the thinking processes they used in making nursing diagnoses. They also tried to clarify the effect of the setting or grouping of clients on the form of those diagnoses and the effects of their conceptual models of nursing on their diagnoses and attendant-thinking processes. The section begins with three chapters written by nurses practicing with clients who have chronic illness. McCorkle describes the diagnostic reasoning process used with people who have terminal cancer; Blainey illustrates the process of arriving at a diagnosis of altered sexuality in persons with diabetes; and Simmons discusses diagnostic reasoning in care of patients with end-stage renal disease. The fourth chapter, by Mitchell, applies the diagnostic process to critically ill persons with neurologic disease.

Each of the contributors operates as a practitioner in a specialized area of practice. Given the structure of the modern health-care system, that specialized area tends to be defined either in terms of setting (for example, intensive care) or disease process of the clientele (for example, diabetes). Consequently, the knowledge-base necessary to determine daily living problems used by each of the contributors is influenced by the setting and the biomedical condition of the group of clients. The biomedical knowledge base is not discussed in this section, even if it is part of the expanded role of the practitioner. Each author was asked to assume that medical diagnoses and management were being competently and concurrently handled so they didn't concern themselves with these factors. Instead, they were asked to focus on the use of data and the knowledge base for management of daily living problems. This difference in focus is exemplified in Chapter 9, where the diagnosis of a critical pathophysiologic state (cardiogenic shock) is discussed as a cue to the nursing diagnosis, *decreased adaptive capacity,* rather than as the end result of the medical-diagnostic process. Each chapter contains illustrative examples of the ways in which medical diagnoses and the knowledge base of pathophysiologic states influence the nursing diagnosis, without becoming the end point of the nursing-diagnostic process.

The chapters are graphic examples of the formative state of our understanding of the diagnostic reasoning processes in nursing, and of the beginning nature of categorization of diagnostic labels. Some chapters categorize the diagnoses broadly; others convey a set of discrete behaviors or symptoms. Still another focuses on the reasoning process in arriving at one category of diagnosis in a given population. All of us began our talks by discussing why we chose certain *actions* (management) in our client populations; and we had to struggle hard to "back up" to the diagnoses that *led* us to the action. This tendency to state interventions rather than diagnosis reflects our educational and action-oriented heritage. It reflects the fact that management in nursing is a more developed art than is diagnosis.

Nonetheless, the commonalities of the thinking process, predicted by Chris Tanner's work, do emerge. To highlight these commonalities, the same set of headings and sequence of presentation are used in each of the chapters. The variations that become evident are in terms of the choice of critical assessment areas, the activators to diagnostic hypotheses, and the influence of setting on the order and urgency of assessment. These similarities and differences will be discussed in the final chapter of the section. Finally, some suggestions will be offered to help the practicing nurse examine a focus and pattern of diagnostic reasoning in her own area of specialized practice.

CHAPTER FIVE

Diagnostic Reasoning in Nursing Care of Advanced Cancer Patients in the Home

Ruth McCorkle

Nursing assessment and diagnosis, as it is used with advanced cancer patients and their families, require high degrees of both sensitivity and flexibility. With the advances in medical technology and specialization, many persons with cancer are living longer with their diseases. As a result, cancer has become recognized primarily as a chronic illness in which the majority of people manage their day-to-day living in their own homes.

From the first contact, whether by phone or in person, the nurse is concerned not only with developing a valid nursing data base and making an accurate nursing diagnosis for effective treatment, but also with developing a climate of reciprocity. In this situation, where the patient is trying to live his daily life effectively while suffering from progressive cancer, a relationship is needed where nurse, patient, and involved family members share mutually in decisions and actions. This style of mutuality profoundly affects the strategies used in gathering data and making decisions as well as in the associated critical thinking engaged in by the nurse involved in their home care. The reader is asked to notice this orientation throughout the chapter.

PRE-ENTRY FACTORS

Effect of the Cancer Care Nursing Specialty

Expertise in cancer-nursing care shapes the initial issues the nurse clinician considers before the initial encounter with a patient or

107

family member occurs. The nature of the neoplastic disease is a primary concern, since differences here create quite different problem areas in daily living.

Solid Tumors.   Solid tumors, particularly in bone, abdomen, and brain, each generate particular problems in daily living that assume significance in the nurse's attention during assessment (McCorkle, 1973). *Bone tumors* create problems of pain management, reduced mobility, and the consequences that these have in all aspects of daily living, including a higher need for readily available physical support services (Catalano, 1981; Donovan, 1976). *Abdominal tumors* quickly affect appetite, nutrition, elimination, and weight changes (losses from anorexia, gains from ascites). Nausea is a frequent source of discomfort (Donovan, 1976). *Brain tumors* require assessment of level of consciousness and orientation, seizure activity, vomiting, vision changes, and loss of other specific functions, together with the impact these have on daily living and the relationships with support figures (Ryan, 1981; Moore, 1981).

Other Tumors.   Where the neoplasms take a form other than solid tumors, the nurse's observation is set to give priority to manifestations of treatment side effects, such as fatigue (secondary to leukopenia), and infections and associate discouragement (Haylock, 1979). The knowledge level regarding the cause of the signs and symptoms is also a priority, *i.e.,* Do the patient and the family know whether the fatigue is caused by a) the treatment and is therefore transient; or b) extension of the disease and is therefore progressive? How accurate are their expectations and goals?

Pre-encounter Patient Data

Unlike some of the other clinical specialities where age, sex, marital status, and other demographic data are seen as significant pre-encounter data affecting the initial data search, these characteristics are less important when the nurse is concerned with how persons are managing their living with advanced cancer. For these patients, the nurse finds essential data prior to a first encounter to include answers to the following questions:

☐ What is the neoplastic diagnosis?
☐ What is the stage of the cancer?
☐ How long ago was the diagnosis made?
☐ Were any difficulties encountered in arriving at the final diagnosis of *cancer?* (*e.g.,* Was the disease

diagnosed first as an inflammatory process before the
cancer was recognized?)

□ How well does the physician who is treating the
cancer know this patient?

□ What is their relationship? (*e.g.*, Has the patient been
referred to a specialist, with whom he or she has had
no previous contact?)

□ Is the patient seen as having credibility by the
health-care providers treating his disease? (*e.g.*, Does
the physician regard the patient as a complainer who
is not taken very seriously?)

Data in these areas influence data-gathering and early diagnosis more
than other aspects of patient data.

Setting-Based Factors

Helping patients manage the impingements imposed by their
disease and treatment side effects in their homes can be constrained
at times due to factors related to the setting. Patients and their family
members maintain control of whom they allow to enter their home
and the frequency of the visits of people who visit. There may be
discrepancies between the nurse and patients' perception of how
often they need to be seen; *e.g.*, bi-monthly, weekly, bi-weekly, or
daily. In addition to the nurse's judgement of how often a patient
needs to be seen, she must plan the frequency of her visits in relation
to the number of patients to be seen, the priority of their problems,
and the geographical location of where they live. The nurse does not
have quick access to the patient's physician and medical records that
are readily available in other settings such as a hospital or clinic. In
order to review a patient's in-hospital or clinic record in planning
care, a release-of-information form must be signed by the patient.
Some patients are reluctant to sign the release form until they are
convinced that home care is needed and that the nurse can help.

It is not uncommon for the nurse to contact a patient's physician
for a symptom-management problem in which medication is needed.
The nurse may attempt to call the physician several times in the same
day, and not reach the physician until sometime the following day.
Then arrangements must be made to have the prescription called to
the patient's pharmacy and the medicine picked up. The process is
more complicated for narcotics because the prescription cannot be a
phone order. Just as time consuming are arrangements the nurse
must make for obtaining supplies and special equipment needed in
the home.

In spite of the limitations imposed by these environmentally related factors, the home setting frequently enhances the nurse's ability to establish a trusting relationship with patients over time. Patients often exhibit a sense of freedom in disclosing pertinent information essential in making decisions, information that is not freely shared in other settings.

ENTRY TO THE DATA FIELD

As noted in the first section of this chapter, the oncology nurse has two goals influencing her behavior as soon as her contact with the patient and family begins. The first goal is to establish a sense of mutual understanding of reciprocity. The patient is responsible for sharing with the nurse facts about his life and how the disease and its treatment impinge on the activities important to him. The nurse is responsible for sharing with the patient her knowledge about questions related to what is happening to the patient and the alternatives available to him. The second goal is to gather a data base that will result in accurate diagnosis and effective treatment of problems in daily living associated with having metastatic cancer. This process must be done within a framework planned with the patient.

Phone Contacts

In this author's community-based practice the first contact is most often initiated by a patient or a relative by telephone, and less frequently by the nurse phoning the patient. However, in either situation, the first priority is to determine the urgency of the presenting situation. How soon do they need or want to be seen by the nurse? Experience shows that both patients and families tend to minimize the urgency of the situation, so it becomes important for the nurse to gather data as to what is actually going on rather than to take the patient's or family's response at face value. Some patients have a great sense of pride and are reluctant to admit they need help.

It is also useful to know, early on, if the patient learned of the home-health services through a physician, a friend, another nurse, or by word of mouth. Knowledge of the referral source can assist in framing the data-gathering approaches. For example, if the patient's physician encouraged the patient to call the nurse, the patient may not recognize the need for home nursing.

Patients and relatives who consult an oncology nurse often do not have a clear idea of what services this kind of a nurse can share with them. As a basis for explaining how this nurse can help them, one needs to know what specific problems they are experiencing. These could be specific problems such as difficulty in breathing or wondering when and how to tell a relative about the situation. On the other hand, they can be diffuse problems such as depression or fatigue. Once the nurse knows what the presenting situation is—what the patient's needs are—it is usually quite simple to spell out clearly what the nurse can do to help.

Face to Face Encounters

The role of social amenities is important in setting the relationship of client and nurse. If the patient comes to be seen at the office, the nurse assumes the role of host as well as health-care provider, making use of social amenities to establish the feeling of reciprocity. These actions include:

walking out of the office to meet the patient and anyone accompanying the patient,

making introductions and using the patient's name,

shaking hands,

asking if they had any difficulty in finding the office,

taking their wraps,

offering seating that is comfortable, and

finding out what time limits they may have on this visit and making them aware of any constraints the nurse may have.

When the nurse goes to the home for the first encounter, the role assumed is that of guest. Here the social amenities are reversed. The nurse

waits to be invited in,

waits to take off her wraps until invited,

asks which chair the patient (host/hostess) usually uses and where they would prefer the nurse to sit.

All of these actions and interactions tell the patient and family that they have control—that the nurse's role is that of helping, not taking over.

Early Areas of Data Collection

Data in a number of areas are important to the nurse who wants to gain knowledge about the patient and his situation early in their relationship in order to maximize the quality of care given. In a chronic progressive illness, the priority of the areas of data gathering are often different than in an acute, short-term illness.

Patient Goals.   The timing of data gathering on patient and family goals is a major area where the nursing assessment tends to vary from other clinical specialities; in acute situations data gathering on patient goals usually occurs late in the assessment. In working with patients with advanced cancer, the issue of patients' goal is addressed in the first meeting in order to foster a sense of client control. The enforced personal and social changes that occur in the life of an ill person as a result of the illness, often necessitate a shift in his life goals. They gradually become more circumscribed.

Clinically, it is important to assess patient goals for two reasons. First, knowledge of the person's goals allows the nurse to quickly assess where the patient is in the process of integrating the meaning of his illness with his life, where he is in understanding his prognosis. Goals allow the nurse to see what the patient's expectations and realities are. For example, if a patient with advanced cancer of the pancreas (who is experiencing jaundice, ascites, and anorexia) wants to return to work, the nurse quickly recognizes that the patient needs additional opportunities to discuss the physical limitations associated with this type of cancer. It may be unrealistic for the patient to return to work and the nurse will expect the patient to eventually exhibit anticipatory grieving behaviors for his potential losses. Secondly, it is essential for the nurse to know the patient's goals so she can help the person accomplish his goals.

There are a number of approaches that are useful in obtaining these data. One may approach this area by saying

> "I need to know what is important to you."
> "We're both hoping that your medical treatment is going
>   to be successful. If it shouldn't work out that way,
>   what would be important to you?"
> "Is there anything you want accomplished?"
> "What do you really want?"
> "How would you like to spend your days?"

If the patient cannot directly address his goals at the initial visit, it is important the nurse initiate the discussion. The nurse can say:

> "Why don't you think about what you really want
> during the time before my next visit. Write down your
> ideas. Then, next time we can talk about them. When
> we both know what's important to you, I can be more
> helpful to you in achieving your goals."

Occasionally, the nurse will encounter a patient who has not thought about his life in relation to certain goals. The nurse needs to be careful not to impose her own expectations on the patient; she needs to work with the patient where he is.

Knowledge of the Disease

It is important for the nurse to observe what the patient and family know about the disease and its implications. Some data will be gathered by direct questioning, for example:

"What are you seeing your doctor for?

What type of treatment has he recommended?

Are you getting any treatments now?

Did he tell you about any side effects you might expect?

What did your doctor say about what to expect from the treatments?"

Other data will be noted through observation, particularly observing the words patients use to refer to the disease, treatment, and prognosis. For example, do they call the disease by name? (*i.e.*, cancer, acute myeloid leukemia) or do they refer to as a mass, a shadow, a lump, arthritis, or lumbago? Do they know the treatment they are receiving or have received by name? Another area that indicates knowledge of the disease is the assessment of the patient's medications. Do they know the names of the medications they are taking? Do they take them as prescribed? When they alter their medication regimen, how and why do they alter it? Do they take extra pills when they feel bad or when they notice a new lump? Do they skip pills when they feel better?

It is important for the nurse to be aware of cues that could indicate sensitive and private issues during her assessment of the patient's health-practicing behaviors. For example, a slight hesitancy on the part of the patient's description of his medications and schedule of administration might indicate that the patient doesn't always adhere to the recommended dosages because of their associated side effects. The nurse needs to give the patient an opportunity to acknowledge the variations he has made in taking his medications in order to live with the side effects without fear of being criticized. Allowing patients to share their own management regimens of the recommended treatments is an important step in establishing a reciprocal and trusting relationship.

Expectations about the disease are often affected by experiences patients have had with others who have had cancer. To assess this the nurse will ask:

"Have you ever known of anyone who had the same disease?" (Was the cancer the same kind, in the same parts of the body?)

"How were they treated?"

"How long ago was this? What was the outcome? What happened to them?"

It is important that the nurse let the patient share his perception of the previous experiences he has had as well as the personal meaning he has developed about cancer and its associated treatments. It is not uncommon for many patients and family members to have misconceptions about the course of their diseases and what to expect. The nurse's acknowledgement of the patient's feelings is essential. It is crucial that she not discredit the information shared. It will take time to assist the patient in understanding what is happening to him and what is not happening.

Support Systems

Many areas of support become crucial in managing daily living with progressing cancer. It eventually becomes important for the nurse to make assessments in many areas of external resources. Human support systems, however, have priority in the initial assessment. The presence of cancer affects and often changes relationships. It is important to know, early on, who is likely to be affected, what the relationships are, if or how they might be expected to change, and what types of personal support systems the patient and family have.

An effective strategy to gather data on the nature of family members and encounters is to use any upcoming holiday as a springboard for this area of data gathering.

"Who are you going to spend Christmas/Thanksgiving/Easter with?"

"Do you usually spend the holiday(s) with your family?"

If there is no holiday in the immediate future, an alternative approach is:

"Do you get together with others for Sunday dinner or for your birthday, anniversary, and so forth?"

Data in these areas of inquiry quickly disclose family-encounter patterns and the members involved.

Family Members' Knowledge
of the Patient's Health Status

Another area of importance is the awareness of family members of the patient's health status. The nurse's concern here is to discover key people who are going to experience difficulty with the change in the patient and his particular disease. For example, parents, regardless of their age or that of their child, always experience more difficulty in losing a child than children do in losing a parent.

The nurse will also want to learn the patient's wishes about involving nuclear- or extended-family members in his situation—the timing and nature of the ill person's wishes for their involvement. If, indeed, the management of daily living is to be collaboratively carried out, the patient's wishes regarding his support system need to be taken into account. The nurse certainly may differ in her views from the patient, and through experience, she may realize that the patient's preferences will create unusual difficulties for both the patient and the family. However the starting point is always the patient's perspective, with negotiations carried out from this base line.

Pets

Pets in the cancer patient's life can be both a resource and a demand. They provide comfort in terms of being a predictable contact with the ill person at any hour of the day and night. However, as the ill persons becomes increasingly dependent, pets can also create additional demands on the caretakers in terms of feeding and care.

Health Care Providers

Health-care providers make up another component of the patient's and family's external resources that need to be a part of the initial assessment. A nurse who is in private practice or who works in a home health-care setting, and thus is seeing patients who are under treatment with other health-care providers, needs information about the patient's perception of his relationships with those providers. This is information that nurses who are employed by hospitals or doctors already tend to have. They frequently know the nature of the patient's and family's relationships with the physicians and the in-patient personnel. If a patient is self-referred to a nurse, or is referred by a non-physician, it becomes important, early on, to gather data on the physician(s) involved in the patient's medical treatment and to learn the patient's perception of the relationships. It is also important to learn how the patient wishes this nurse to relate to the physician(s) involved in his care. Data here can be gathered by asking:

"What doctors are you seeing?"

"How long have you been seeing them?"

"Do you find it easy to talk with them?"

"I can meet your needs best if I talk with your physician(s) on a regular basis. How do you wish me to work with them on your behalf?"

At times, the physician(s) involved in the patient's treatment are known to the nurse. The nurse is able to provide more efficient care to the patient if she has knowledge of how each physician practices, for example, whether he shares his practice with others, how available he is by phone, what his on-call schedule is, and so forth. Over time, the nurse knows which physician will medicate for pain but not for anxiety, and which will medicate for anxiety but not for pain. She learns which physician listens to the patient's goals, which one accords credibility to patients' reports, and which one treats cancer aggressively and for how long when the prognosis grows graver. All of these areas of knowledge are important if the nurse is to collaborate with the patient and physician in order to effectively help the patient manage that part of daily living concerned with incorporating the biomedical treatment. When the physician, his treatment, and his practice patterns are not known to the nurse, the nurse needs to gather these data to integrate with the patient-family data base. The same is true where other health-care providers are involved—other nurses (inpatient or clinic nurses), social workers, chaplains, and so on.

Environmental Supports and Barriers

Environmental supports and barriers are also elements of the patient data base and can be crucial elements in planning care as the patient's internal resources are depleted by disease or treatment. A home visit yields a wealth of data concerning both resources and barriers in the environment. The nurse can be a realist in planning with the patient and primary family-care-givers about management of daily living only when there is accurate data on stairs, space, distances to bathroom, utilities, phone and transportation—the physical elements that form a basic foundation to daily living.

Physical Status

The patient's physical status is of course basic to all decision making about management of daily living. While other data are being gathered verbally, the nurse is making observations regarding the patient's physical status. These observations include noticing:

Is the patient dressed?

What is the status of grooming?

Does the person move about without signs of discomfort or dysfunction?

Does speech seem normal? Any breaks in sentences due to shortness of breath? Is there more sighing than normal?

What is the patient's affect? Does the patient seem to respond appropriately with different cues; for example, does the patient smile when a compliment is offered or does the patient demean the acknowledgement.

Patterns of Activities and Demands in Daily Living

The nurse also needs information on the usual or preferred patterns in daily living in addition to any adjustments patients are having to make. Here the approach could be: "Tell me what your usual day is like. Start with what time you get up; when you eat, dress, and so on." As they discuss the day, ask about what feels "okay" to them and what is troublesome.

The critical thinking the nurse engages in here is to try to associate which activities or changes in activities are creating difficulties. For example, Mrs. Larson, who was suffering from breast cancer with bone metastasis, was managing well all day except for the homecoming of the son and husband at suppertime. She became very discouraged as she shared her increased feelings of frustration and failure with the nurse. She perceived herself as being no more active prior to supper than at other times of the day. However, when the nurse pursued more detail on the amount of activity involved in planning supper, such as the number of steps she was taking, the source of the problem became obvious. She was walking more and moving more in the process of cooking and getting supper on the table. Strengthening the pain cocktail for that period of the day solved the difficulty so she could remain active doing the things she wanted and enjoy the time with her family.

Patient Role in Ongoing Assessment

Once the major areas of strength and dysfunction have been delineated and integrated with the patterns of daily living and goals in the initial assessment, ongoing monitoring and fine-tuning of the nursing diagnoses continue. Again, the goal is mutual participation of the client and nurse. A very useful technique, it has been found, is the patient-kept log.

The nurse, based on her preliminary assessment, identifies the categories where daily monitoring and documentation would seem productive. The patient confirms or modifies them. Decisions are made as to the most productive times, intervals, and durations for monitoring as well as the unit of measurement (such as number of steps, minutes of activity, pulse rate, duration of relief from pain, rest times needed to regain energy, amount of food taken, and so forth). Patients with identical diagnoses usually end up with differing log categories because of the differences in response to the disease/status of treatment or activities, and because of the demands of daily living and the environment for their specific daily life. Thus the nurse does not use a standard log form, but determines the elements of the log and the units of measure based on data from each patient's presenting situation. She also modifies it as conditions change. An example of a log format used for a patient with breast cancer and bone metastasis can be found in the lists on the following page.

The patient has the role of contributing to the categories and refining the units of measure as the log is set up. Beyond that, his responsibility is to engage in the planned self-monitoring and record the findings. (An assessment log is found in Table 5-1.)

Together, the patient and nurse evaluate the findings and determine from them the management strategies that would seem most productive. The findings are also used in making contacts with the physician for alterations in medical treatment. Most physicians appreciate a documented systematic data base illustrating changes in patients' symptoms and treatment responses.

Bringing Closure in Initial Assessment

When either the time available for the assessment transaction has ended or the interaction is completed, definitive closure is needed. The findings of strengths and effective management of daily living as well as limitations, dysfunctions, and associated problems in daily living, are summarized by the nurse in an organized fashion. The patient is encouraged to participate with both validation or modifications. The nurse asks the patient directly:

"Is that the way you see it?"

"Is that the way it is?"

CATEGORIES OF ASSESSMENT FOR PATIENT LOG*

Daily Activities
Bathing
Toileting
Dressing
Walking
Stair-climbing
Cooking
Driving
Working
Lifting/Twisting
· Groceries
· Wash

Personal Patterns
Diet
· Type
· Frequency of Meals
· Favorite Foods
· Roughage Foods
Bowel
· Type of stool
· Frequency
· Cathartics
Appearance
· Hair
· Nails
Sleep
· Length/Wakefulness
· Frequency
· Medications

Socialization with Others
Spouse
· Type of Activity
· Frequency
Family Members
Neighbors
Work Associates
Church Members
Other

Common Symptoms
Pain
· Location
· Pattern/Type
· Frequency
· What aggravates it
· Amount of weight-bearing
· Interventions
· Medications
Fatigue
· Characteristics
· Periods of Rest
· Diet
· Type of activities
· Associated other symptoms, *e.g.,* sleep
Mood

* These categories are recommended for consideration of a woman with breast cancer with metastasis to bones, *e.g.,* vertebra, pelvis, femur. The patient would not be asked to record data in all categories but only one or two in which the patient and nurse together have identified that they need additional data.

Finally the expectations for what each person will do during the interval before the next contact are made explicit; such as "the patient will maintain the log as agreed and will undertake whatever activities have been decided upon." Conditions under which the patient is to contact the nurse are agreed upon. The nurse either will or will not contact the physician; she will review the medical records, or do whatever has been negotiated. Thus the activity of closure includes both what has taken place and future expectations of role relationships and activities for each party. Each activity has been verbally and explicitly dealt with.

COMMONLY ACTIVATED GENERATED DIAGNOSTIC HYPOTHESES WITH ADVANCED CANCER PATIENTS

In medicine, students are taught to retrieve common diagnostic possibilities associated with the pattern of presenting cues as part of the diagnostic reasoning process. They are also taught to consider uncommon problems as well, such as those infrequently occurring diagnoses that, if present, can produce significant consequences. The same pattern of generating diagnostic hypotheses is useful in the oncology nurse's diagnostic reasoning.

Common diagnostic categories to consider with advanced cancer patients include:

Dysfunction in daily living secondary to pain, (Anderson, 1982)

Dysfunction in daily living secondary to fatigue, (Krant, 1981)

Malnutrition and loss of life satisfaction associated with eating and food-related social events, (Butler, 1980)

Unsatisfying relationships with family member(s), (Maxwell, 1981)

Unsatisfying or ineffective relationships with health-care provider(s), (Krant, 1977–1978)

Loss of control over segments of one's life—emotional, decision-making, physical, (Greenwald and Nevitt, 1982)

or

Loss of independence in areas seen by the patient as crucial (Lewis, 1982).

Problems that do not occur so often, but which carry high risk and therefore need to be considered include:

The solitary person—the one who lives alone. The independent person who has studiously avoided need for external personal resources, and the social isolate or deviant. Such persons are at risk for problems in managing daily living with advancing cancer because they eventually will have to depend on others. They do not have the skills associated with dependency and they have few personal support persons "in the wings." Achieving satisfaction, or even managing daily living for these people as the disease progresses, is very chancey under these conditions.

Each of these areas of discomfort or dysfunction in daily living are common enough, or urgent enough, to recommend regular consideration by the nurse as she generates hypotheses from the presenting situation.

DIAGNOSIS-DIRECTED DATA SEARCH

Each of the diagnostic categories, when retrieved in response to a presenting-patient situation, should bring to mind an observational guide that directs the nurse's subsequent search in the data field to the end that an accurate definitive diagnosis is made. Two major diagnostic categories will be used to illustrate the diagnosis-directed data search.

Pain and Daily Living

When the patient presents with the manifestations of pain, there may be noticeable changes in the person's appearance and personal habits of grooming. Patients in pain move more slowly, accomplish less, and can be easily irritated. In addition, the patient has frequently learned "to pass" with his pain so he does not appear different (Benoliel et al., 1980). For example, patients learn quickly that pain is not a socially accepted topic of discussion and health-care professionals are not very responsive to chronic complainers. Patients want to say little to alienate themselves from others. Often, patients do not verbalize directly their complaints of pain, but rather talk about activities they are no longer able to do. It is important for the nurse to be aware of the fact that many patients are reluctant to use the word "pain" and therefore may deny its presence, because of the stigma associated with it. Additional observations about the impact of this pain and its associated dysfunction should be made in terms of the following areas:

- [ ] What activities and demands of daily living affect the pain? Do they make it worse or better?
- [ ] What activities and demands of daily living are most impacted upon by the presence of pain? What alterations have been made because of the pain? How satisfied is the client and how are others affected by the alterations?
- [ ] How are others in his immediate daily living environment responding to the patient's pain? How is it affecting their daily living?
- [ ] What are the patient's verbal and nonverbal manifestations of pain? Are they congruent? How does the cultural background of the patient affect the way this person communicates his pain and suffering? Do the patient's patterns of communicating pain and suffering achieve effective or counterproductive responses from others, such as family and health care providers? Do the responses of others enhance or detract from the patient's sense of well-being and credibility?
- [ ] What is the natural history of the pain? What is the organic reference for this pain, *e.g.*, bone metastasis, pressure . . .?

An example of a nurse's data-gathering and differential diagnosis associated with pain may prove useful to the reader.

Mrs. Marion has a diagnosis of *primary breast tumor* that was treated with mastectomy and chemotherapy. Several years later she now has boney metastasis. Radiation has been used. She still has sufficient pain to require the use of a pain cocktail, oral morphine. The cocktail has been controlling the pain so that she can manage the homemaking activities of daily living in collaboration with her husband and a son in his late teens. Today she calls in great distress, asking that her pain cocktail be increased in strength because it is no longer controlling the pain.

The nurse is familiar with the progress of the disease in this patient and believes there is no organic basis for the increased pain at this point. She asks, "Has anything been going on in your daily living that could increase your pain? Are you doing anything different?" Mrs. Marion can think of no change in physical activity—only that the pain is so much worse today and she is anxious and depressed by it. The nurse inquires further, "Has *anything* changed at home for you? Well . . . yes," is the hesitant reply, "my husband has been losing so much sleep because of my restlessness at night that his job has been suffering. Last night he moved out of our double bed and the bedroom we've shared for all of the twenty years of our marriage."

The nurse had worked enough with the husband to know that he is devoted to his wife. She also knows that he has a very responsible and demanding position and that he is a light sleeper. She is aware that sleep deprivation had been a growing problem for Mr. Marion in recent weeks.

For the patient, the nurse's diagnosis was that *her suffering had been increased, not by the cancer, but by the loss of her husband's presence near her during the night,* and also the possible rejection she was experiencing secondary to the symbolism of her husband's move from the bed they had shared. Her nights were wakeful and long; his presence and all it symbolized had been a source of comfort. The loneliness and anxiety related to loss and possible rejection were compounding the existing pain. For the husband, the nurse's diagnosis was sleep deprivation and fatigue—not rejection of his chronically ill wife. Treatment needed to be directed toward the patient's self concept as a wife and the husband's need for respite so that both could function optimally, individually and together. This is quite a different diagnosis and treatment plan than one dealing merely with increased pain.

Fatigue and Daily Living

Fatigue is a diagnostic category to be activated when the following clues are present. The nurse observes that the patient talks less and sighs more. Similar to many of the behaviors expressed by the patient in pain, the person moves more slowly and his personal appearance declines. The patient no longer dresses, shaving is neglected, hair is not combed or cared for as it was. Irritability increases, the patient is short with people. The person's orientation shifts from an other-oriented to self-oriented. The person freely acknowledges that he is tired, and no matter how much rest he gets, he continually wakes up tired. The tiredness is also associated with other related symptoms such as a lack of appetite and constipation. The patient expresses feelings of heaviness of his head, his body, and legs. He yawns frequently and wants to lie down.

Fatigue is closely related to nutrition. Fatigue may either cause poor nutrition because the patient is too tired to shop, cook, or eat; or, it may be caused directly by poor nutrition. Thus the diagnosis may be:

Fatigue → inadequate food intake secondary to no energy for shopping for food, preparing food, or eating food prepared by others

or

Inadequate food intake 2° anorexia or the desire to die more quickly → depression manifested as fatigue.

Since each of these diagnoses would be treated somewhat differently, it becomes critical to direct the data search in such a way that an accurate differential diagnosis is made.

Further, fatigue in itself, whether it is the result of or cause of inadequate food and fluid intake, impacts on daily living in predictable areas and in significant ways. Thus, secondary diagnoses delineating the effects on daily living are also crucial to appropriate nursing management. A diagnosis of fatigue should direct the nurse's data search to determine:

changes in sleep patterns (increase in insomnia is
   common),

degree of understanding of what is happening,

effect on ability to evacuate the bowel,

effect on eating and desire to eat,

effect on interpersonal relationships and social activities,
   and

effect on person's self-esteem and sense of personal
   worth

An example of a man experiencing increased fatigue follows.

Mr. Boon had a diagnosis of *rectal cancer* several years ago and underwent an abdominal–perineal resection. His physicians were hopeful they had cured Mr. Boon until six months ago, when he was admitted with a small bowel obstruction. At that time, he again underwent surgery to relieve the obstruction and received postoperative radiation to reduce the tumor. Three months later, a specialist recommended that he take chemotherapy. Gradually, over the last two months, Mr. Boon has continued to lose weight and has subsequently lost interest in his personal appearance. The chemotherapy has made him leukopenic and anemic. His appetite has been nonexistent and he has little energy to interact with others. He has become very discouraged because he doesn't seem to improve. When questioned about what is happening to him, Mr. Boon has little knowledge about the side effects of his cancer therapies and the symptoms related to the progression of his cancer. He believes if he could just eat he could get his strength back and he wouldn't be so tired.

For the patient, the nurse's diagnosis was that *much of Mr. Boon's feelings of fatigue were directly related to his physiological changes induced by the cancer therapies secondary to his ability to eat the necessary dietary foods he needs.*

It can be seen that the prevailing pattern in the diagnostic-reasoning process, of first activating general diagnostic hypotheses and then moving to generate more specific associated diagnoses, is used in this nursing specialty also. The diagnostician first identifies the major categories of cancer-related dysfunction and then moves on to the more specific forms that the dysfunction can take on, together with the areas of impact on activities and demands of daily living.

HYPOTHESIS TESTING

Evaluation of diagnostic hypotheses seems to proceed almost concurrently with the continuing activation process. First the nurse compares the presenting patient data with the characteristics associated with the *general* diagnostic category, such as pain, fatigue, loneliness, and fear. When there is a match here, then she uses the cues in the patient situation to activate the more precise diagnostic possibilities. An example of such a distinction would be the nurse's judgment in making a diagnosis that Mrs. Marion's *pain was increased by the perceived loss of her husband's physical presence at night* contrasted with Mrs. Larson, whose diagnosis was *bone pain increases associated with increased physical activity at the supper hour.*

PROGNOSTIC VARIABLES FOR DAILY LIVING WITH PROGRESSIVE CANCER

Determination of a prognosis for managing daily living with progressive cancer is as crucial to effective nursing management as the pathophysiologic prognosis is to biomedical management of the neoplastic process. An important insight for practitioners in the two major disciplines involved in the care of most cancer patients is that the two prognoses are not identical, nor are they fully dependent upon each other. They can vary independently of one another.

Differences between Biomedical and Nursing Prognoses in Progressive Cancer

With advanced cancer, the biomedical prognosis is obviously poor, the trajectory is downward, the outcome, ultimately, is death. The only questions are the time lines and the severity of physiological problems en route.

The nursing prognosis on the other hand can have a more positive outcome. Daily living can be effective, relationships rewarding, completed tasks can provide a sense of accomplishment, and all this despite progressing disease. The quality of life can contine to be satisfying, even as it is changing.

The biomedical and nursing perspectives are different. The variables upon which they are based are different. Therefore the outcomes can be expected to be different—even though the prognoses for each specialty are similar.

This is not to say that alterations in each aspect of the patients' situation do not affect the other. Gains in control of the disease and symptoms obviously make the management of daily living and all its ramifications easier. Conversely, medical-treatment failure or failure in palliation can complicate daily living. By the same token, effectiveness in managing daily living and positive interaction between the patient and those closely involved can enhance response to treatment. So, each component of patient response affects, but does not control, the other.

Patients with advanced cancer almost uniformly die of the disease; their families experience loss and grief. Yet many patients and families experience a "good" death and personal growth in the process. Nurses engaged in calculating patient prognosis need to consider these relationships in their thinking.

Prognostic Variables

What are the prognostic variables the nurse considers when arriving at an accurate picture for the patient with progressing cancer. In broad categories they will concern: 1) the internal resources the patient brings to the situation, 2) the external resources available to the patient—their stability and goodness of fit to the patient's needs, and 3) opportunities for personal satisfaction and growth in the course of living out the days and weeks.

Internal Resource Variables.   The nurse will want data on the following areas concerned with status of internal resources:

- ☐ Which signs and symptoms of the cancer or its treatment are being effectively managed? Which are not?
- ☐ Are there ways to compensate for those signs and symptoms that are not being controlled so as to minimize their impact on daily living? How important to the patient are the ADLs and DDLs, and how are they affected by the dysfunction? What kinds of accomodations can or will the patient make in activities or demands of daily living? Will the quality of life still be satisfying to the patient?

External Resource Variables.   External resources that affect prognosis for the advanced cancer patient include people (both personal and professional networks) and nonhuman resources, such as money, medications, home environment, transportation, and diversion, among others.

Data are needed regarding external resources in the following areas:

- ☐ Is there one consistent person the patient can count on to stay close and stick by him regardless of the course of events?
- ☐ Is there a support network to provide respite for the primary support figure and primary care giver(s)?
- ☐ Is the primary physician supportive of the patient's goals in the treatment of the disease and of the patient's style of living with his cancer? Is the physician available and approachable?
- ☐ If the patient must be hospitalized, are the nurses

supportive of the patient's goals and lifestyle? Is there one among them ready and able to assume the role of primary nurse to coordinate the planned care?

☐ Is there money available for food, supplies, medications, phone calls, other utilities, and any extra equipment needed?

Opportunities for Personal Satisfaction and Growth

Illness affords people an opportunity to review the meaning of their lives and to identify what is personally important to them. In the day-to-day living with the impingements resulting from cancer and its associated treatments, patients need assistance in establishing short-term goals and bench marks in order to see their accomplishments. Patients who demonstrate positive attitudes seem to live longer and cope better with their diseases. It has been common practice for nurses to assess the problem areas related to that which the person and his family are experiencing, and not to emphasize the strengths that emerge when patients are facing changes imposed by their illness. Nurses can frequently obtain a great deal of satisfaction in helping patients to interpret the positive aspects of their illness and to achieve the short-term goals that have been mutually established. Data are needed in the following areas:

☐ What does life mean to the person?

☐ How has the person's meaning of life changed since his illness?

☐ Have there been any benefits to the illness; what have they been?

SUMMARY

In this chapter, the process of assessment and the identification of nursing problems for patients with advanced cancer have been presented. In order to advance nursing practice, two things are needed: a systematic approach by nurses for data gathering and a common recognition that the areas of focus of assessment are the essential content base for helping patients manage with advanced cancer. There are differences among nursing specialists as to the priority of patient problems. Mundinger identifies three broad categories of patient responses useful for formulating nursing diagnoses for cancer patients: voluntary physical; involuntary physical, and nonphysical;

and psychological and emotional (Mundinger, 1978). In community-health nursing, the nurse needs to let the patient be the leader in establishing the areas of priorities and formulating the diagnostic categories.

The state of the art in cancer nursing, as in other specialty areas that specify diagnostic characteristics associated with daily living and dysfunction, is still in its infancy—formal, standardized nursing diagnoses and criteria really do not exist. However, within the knowledge base and experience of clinical experts who deal regularly with advanced cancer patients, informal diagnoses and reliable criteria really are known. Problem recognition takes place based on evaluation, and nursing diagnoses are applied. The diagnostic-reasoning process takes place, even if on an informal basis. This chapter is an initial step in formalizing this process.

Table 5–1

Example of Log for Assessment of Daily Routine for Woman with Breast Cancer and Bone Metastasis

Identified Areas of Concern by Patient and Nurse

Increasing Pain, Poor Appetite, and Fatigue

Instructions to Patient

For five days, record the following:
When you get up
How you feel
What activities you do
When and what you eat
Family and friend contacts
When you go to bed
How you sleep

Patient Entry for Day One

Time	Activity	Patient Intervention
7 a.m.	Unable to get out of bed in morning. Irritable, yelling at son to get to school.	Takes two codeine tablets.
8 a.m.	Gets out of bed—sleepy, no desire to get dressed. Husband leaves for work. No desire to eat, picks at breakfast.	Takes a nap at 8:30 a.m.

(continued on next page)

Table 5–1 (*continued*)

Example of Log for Assessment of Daily Routine for Woman with Breast Cancer and Bone Metastasis

Patient Entry for Day One

Time	Activity	Patient Intervention
9:30 a.m.	Gets up; washes and dresses, begins preparation for dinner. Reads. Interacts with neighbor.	
12:30 p.m.	Eats lunch. Walks dog using a cane.	Takes one codeine tablet.
3:30 p.m.	Son comes home from school.	
4:30 p.m.	Prepares dinner. Increased pain, irritable.	Takes one codeine tablet.
5:00 p.m.	Husband home—dinner on table—unable to eat, nauseous	Takes a nap at 5:30 p.m.
6:30 p.m.	Helps clean up dishes. Watches TV with husband, reads paper.	
9 p.m.	Gets ready for bed.	Takes one codeine tablet.
10 p.m.	Goes to bed, sleeps, exhausted.	
2 a.m.	Up to bathroom. Able to go back to sleep, still tired.	

Preliminary Nursing Diagnosis

Chronic fatigue and inadequate nutrition secondary to inadequate pain management increased physical activity and weight bearing throughout the day and increased the patient's pain; as a result, patient medicated herself for pain. Blood level of narcotic needed to be maintained, rather than patient experiencing peaks and valleys from narcotic.

Nursing Intervention

Nurse validates with patient interpretation made based on observations. Teach patient about pattern of pain and the need to medicate self before pain becomes troublesome. Have patient medicate self on a regular four-hour basis and particularly take pain medicine one hour prior to time scheduled to get out of bed in morning. Continue to monitor pain pattern and the effectiveness of drug that is ordered, especially to rule out progression of cancer and need for medical treatment.

Change log entries to include data on specific location of pain, type and pattern of pain, and what relieves pain. Patient to continue log entries for next 4 days.

BIBLIOGRAPHY

McCorkle MR: Coping with Physical Symptoms in Metastatic Breast Cancer. American Journal of Nursing 73:1034–1038, 1973

Catalano RB: Supportive Care of the Seriously Ill Cancer Patient: Control of Pain. In Oncologic Emergencies edited by Yarbro JW and Bornstein RS. New York. Grune and Stratton, 1981

Donovan MI and Pierce SG: Cancer Care Nursing. pp. 44–92 NY: Appleton-Century-Crofts, 1976

Donovan MI and Pierce SG: Nutrition in Cancer Care Nursing, pp. 130–155 NY: Appleton-Century-Crofts, 1976

Ryan LS: Nursing Assessment of the Ambulatory Patient with Brain Metastases. Cancer Nursing, 4:281–291, 1981

Moore P: Safety problems encountered by clients with brain tumors. In Cancer Nursing, pp. 582–594. Edited by L. Marino. St. Louis: The C.V. Mosby Company, 1981

Haylock PJ and Hart LK: "Fatigue in patients receiving localized radiation," Cancer Nursing, 2:461–467, 1979

Anderson JL: Nursing Management of the Cancer Patient in Pain: A Review of the Literature. Cancer Nursing, 5:33–41, 1982

Krant MJ and Roy PF: "Psychologic Exigencies in Oncology" in Oncologic Emergencies, edited by J.W. Yarbro and R.S. Bornstein. New York: Grune and Stratton, 1981, pp. 395–409

Butler JH: Nutrition and Cancer: A Review of the Literature. Cancer Nursing, 3:131–136, 1980

Maxwell MB: Cancer, Hypoalbuminemia, and Nutrition. Cancer Nursing, 4:451–458, 1981

Krant MJ and Johnston L: Family Members' Perceptions of Communications in Late Stage Cancer. International Journal of Psychiatry in Medicine, 8:203–216, 1977–78

Greenwald HP and Nevitt MC: Physician Attitudes Toward Communication with Cancer Patients, Social Science and Medicine, 16:59–594, 1982

Lewis FM: Experienced Personal Control and Quality of Life in Late-Stage Cancer Patients. Nursing Research, 31:113–119, 1982

Benoliel JQ, McCorkle R and Young K: Development of a Social Dependency Scale. Research in Nursing and Health, 3:3–10, 1980

Goffman E: Stigma. Englewood Cliffs, N.J.: Prentice Hall, Inc. 1963

Mundinger MO: Nursing Diagnoses for Cancer Patients. Cancer Nursing, 1:221–226, 1978

CHAPTER SIX

Diagnostic Reasoning in Nursing Management of Persons with End-Stage Renal Disease on Dialysis

Gail P. Simmons

Chronic renal failure and its biomedical treatment create pervasive and difficult problems in managing daily living. Living to promote health and minimize the deficits produced by the disease and its treatment requires careful nursing diagnosis and management that involves patients, their families, and their environments.

The components of the diagnostic reasoning process as they are used in this clinical nursing specialty, chronic renal failure, will be discussed in this chapter. *Patterns* of thinking—the common problems that need to be considered and the critical areas of data to be taken into consideration—will be illustrated. Beyond this, the reader will need to determine how *specific data* in a given patient situation at a particular point in time will generate the *individual diagnosis* for that patient.

PRE-ENTRY FACTORS

Factors that influence the nurse's thinking even before the first patient encounter include the nursing specialty area, specific patient data, the stage of medical treatment, and the clinical environment.

Effect of the Renal Nursing Specialty

Expertise in physiology, pathophysiology, biomedical management of renal disease, and regular nursing care of a clientele with this

133

pathology tends to result in a mind-set that causes one to look for responses and risks in areas of daily living particularly affected. These problem areas include diet, fluids, fatigue, sleep, change in body image, constraints on mobility, and status of support systems. Problems in these areas of daily living occur so regularly with this patient population that they tend to become an important focus in nursing assessment and diagnosis with these patients and their families. This focus on a particular group of problems may tend to bias the way in which data are collected and used. It also may tend to blind the renal nurse specialist to cues indicating problems that do not fall within these categories.

Pre-encounter Patient Data

There are certain pieces of data about a patient that tend to modify the direction of nursing assessment. This data collection can take place even before one actually sees the patient.

Age, Sex, and Marital Status.   Age, sex, and marital status suggest both strength and areas of high risk. For example: a *young male* tends to have greater difficulty adhering to the dietary regimen. *Older males,* particularly those who have been married for many years, will often have the help of wives who are willing to prepare food in appropriate ways. *Young or middle-aged women* are at greater risk of losing the support of their spouses or partners.

Names.   Names linked to certain cultural backgrounds suggest the likelihood that high usual sodium content in the diet may be difficult if not impossible to change. Another cultural factor among certain groups is the existence and importance of extended family. This family's network and its relationships can influence the patient's decision making, self-concept, and social life as he attempts to manage daily living with renal failure.

Addresses.   Addresses suggest kinds of neighborhoods, affluence, types of housing (apartments, rooms, single-family dwellings), transportation, and accessibility of treatment and professional resources. The nature of the home environment can be particularly important if home dialysis is being considered.

Stage of Medical Treatment.   Has the client been treated as an outpatient with declining renal function for a period of months or years, or has the onset of renal failure been more sudden and acute, *i.e.,* as a result of trauma, cancer? The amount/extent of exposure that each client has had with his or her illness will influence the direction of nursing assessment. Additional medical diagnoses or pathology suggest additional risk factors. For example pre-existing diabetes suggests the risks of visual deficits and circulatory disorders, which would complicate daily living with renal disease.

Summary. As important as each of these units of data may be in accurately and efficiently diagnosing the patient's problems in daily living, the nurse must be careful and only allow them to raise questions, not predetermine diagnoses. Premature interpretation of such information or any stereotyping may lead one to make inaccurate inferences with subsequent data and also close off important avenues of data gathering. Pre-encounter data can and should be used, but carefully.

Factors in the Environment that Influence the Assessment Process

For patients with chronic renal failure, the home environment and family are crucial elements in the patient's successful management of daily living with end-stage renal disease. If nurses are making assessments and treating the patient in a clinical work setting where there is no access to direct observation of the home environment and family, they will have to depend on the patient's perceptions, and these may or may not be valid. Where nurses cannot go to the home or meet with the family, it becomes important to have a specific approach to assessment of these aspects of the data base so that factual, objective data are available as well as subjective data of patient feelings.

ENTRY TO THE DATA FIELD

The data base the nurse needs in order to effectively diagnose and treat the problems in daily living that are encountered by patients with end-stage renal disease incorporates both concrete facts and sensitive, feeling-oriented considerations. Certain strategies have been found to be useful in helping the patient to comfortably and effectively share his data.

Because end-stage renal disease affects almost every element of daily living, a logical and usually comfortable place to start is with the daily routine. The nurse may say, "Tell me what a typical day was like for you before you became sick." When the patient has given this information, the nurse may then progress to, "Describe what a typical day and night are like for you now."

Nutrition is a critical area widely affected by both the disease and its treatment. Here again, a useful approach is to gather data on previous eating habits and current patterns. One also needs information such as: what are the patterns of eating out, who does the shopping for food, who does the cooking, and how many persons are regularly present for meals (Note: adherence to the diet is made more difficult if the person eats alone or with a number of persons who don't wish to be inhibited by the patient's diet).

By starting with concrete areas of inquiry, the nurse frequently gets cues and indications of the more sensitive psychosocial aspects that can then be addressed in an individualized manner using data the patient has already shared.

ACTIVATION OF DIAGNOSTIC HYPOTHESES

Diagnostic hypotheses in patients with end-stage renal disease are activated from certain major categories of data that are routinely assessed on all patients and families. These categories encompass the major areas of nursing diagnoses, as shown in the list below.

Common Nursing Diagnostic Categories in End-Stage Renal Disease

Adherence to Diet Modifications
Fatigue
Sleep Disturbance
Support Systems
Attitude Toward Time
Recognition of Change in Body Response to ADL
Mobility Restriction
Body Image
Denial
Restricted Ability to Learn

The categories of data from which nursing diagnoses are commonly derived include all of the contents of the list.

Diet and Potential Problems in Diet Modifications

Risk Factors. As mentioned earlier, certain age groups, sex and marital statuses, as well as living situations tend to suggest greater risks of problems in managing daily living in the area of diet modification. The young single male has often shown difficulty in adhering to the dietary regimen. Persons eating in large family groups may have difficulty in getting the dietary modifications needed, particularly if the person doing the cooking has difficulty in understanding or accepting the differences. Obviously the shopping and cooking skills of the person preparing the food are going to influence the patient's success in managing diet and the degree of satisfaction found in the food he eats. Patterns of eating out also influence adherence to dietary restrictions. Persons whose occupation or lifestyle require them to eat out often, will find sodium restrictions difficult to control.

Where the cultural food patterns normally incorporate high-sodium content, there is of course greater risk in gaining adherence to a low-sodium diet. Here the attitudes of family, for or against adherence, can also be a major factor.

Where other diseases also have dietary regimens it may be difficult to achieve a balance between the two, often opposing, needs. For example, if a person has emphysema and adequate hydration is needed to liquefy the chest secretions, while at the same time the renal diet requires fluid restrictions, the patient is in a double bind. Which dietary requirement takes precedence? Is a balance possible?

Manifestations of Dietary Problems.   The signs and symptoms of failure to manage the dietary patterns effectively tend to emerge fairly quickly. The nurse will see extreme changes in fluid weight gain within a 1 to 3 day interval. Potassium values will be persistently high. The patient will report a "poor appetite" for the "new" foods. There will also be complaints of extreme thirst.

Fatigue and Implications
for Activities of Daily Living

Fatigue is a persistent and regular problem facing the individual with end-stage renal disease. It results both from the low hematocrits and the failure of the body to excrete the toxic wastes.

Risk Factors.   Fatigue will tend to be a more major nursing management problem when certain conditions exist. If the present work demands and daily activities are perceived by the patient as either crucial or highly desirable, fatigue and inability to maintain the desired lifestyle will be particularly troublesome. This is true also when the patient has major family responsibilities and sees no acceptable surrogate to share or take over the work load. At times, an active social life and entertainment schedule is seen as necessary for the preferred lifestyle. Here too, fatigue will be a source of major dissatisfaction.

Fatigue will tend to be influenced by the hematocrit baseline at which the patient finally settles, by the feedback cycle. Generally speaking, if the hematocrit stabilizes at above 20%, the client will be able to function well although stamina will be greatly reduced unless the hematocrit becomes stabilized at greater than 27%. Fatigue is of course also influenced by other medical complications as well as the energy that is required for prescribed exercise regimens introduced into the daily living by the physician. If the supply of energy is limited, any energy that is used for a prescribed exercise regimen will not be available for activities the patient might rather engage in—hence there are risks of patient dissatisfaction or possibly noncompliance.

Manifestations.   The manifestations of fatigue tend to occur in the form of reports by the patient that they have no "staying power" for any kind of extended physical activity. "I feel tired all the time" is a common subjective complaint. There may also be complaints of inability to "maintain any kind of social life." The nurse may also note more shortness-of-breath with ambulation within the clinical setting or dialysis unit.

Sleep Disturbances and Usual Management of Sleep Loss

Risk Factors.   Factors that increase risk of sleep disturbances are associated with previous lifestyle as well as with the current alterations. Age is a factor; for instance, older persons experience more sleep disturbances normally and are thus at greater risk. Past patterns of stress disrupting sleep increase the risks of sleep disruption with end-stage renal disease and with dialysis treatment. Dependence on chemical sleep-aids in the past also increases risks, reflecting as it does the patient's previous dissatisfaction with sleep patterns.

The current health status and its treatment creates risks of sleep disruption. Anemia contributes to insomnia. The creation of permanent blood access via cannula, fistula, or catheter often creates stress, as patients are afraid to fall asleep for fear the channel will open and they will bleed to death. "Restless Leg Syndrome," or nocturnal leg cramps, can greatly disturb sleep. The dialysis itself can disrupt the management of sleep problems. When the dialysis is scheduled for the daytime, the patient spends increased time in a chair or bed during the day—with increased opportunities for napping. Further, if the dialysis is scheduled in the early morning hours, it may occur just as the person is able to move into a sound sleep after a sleepless night.

Manifestations. Sleep disruption will often result in direct complaints of insomnia to the nurse combined with requests for sleeping pills. One may see patterns of lateness for early morning appointments. Patients may report or may be seen sleeping in the daytime. They may indicate that they are afraid to go to sleep because of the fear of bleeding from the cannula. They may also report increasing irritability.

Status of Support System

Risk Factors. Strengths or risk factors will be associated with a variety of conditions. Marital status, the strength of the nuclear or extended family, closeness of bonds between friends and partners are all major strengths and or risks when one considers the need for support and a permanently changed lifestyle. Age is also a factor.

The nature and strength of one's religious beliefs and affiliations are variables that affect support systems, both internal and external. For example, a belief against blood transfusions creates real complications in a disease and treatment that results in ongoing anemia.

Cultural factors affect dietary practices, decision making, social life, and many aspects of the way a patient participates in the health care regimen. The economic impact of the disease and its treatment on the individual, the family and lifestyle cannot be ignored. Chronic disease, particularly one treated with high technology over the rest of the person's lifetime, is a tremendous financial drain. How the family deals with these factors contributes to the risks or strengths in managing daily living.

The patient's family's educational background, previous contacts with the health care system, and capacity to understand the disease, the treatment and the health-care system all contribute to the family members' capacities to use support systems effectively or not.

Geographic location (rural/suburban/urban) gives rise to examination of risk factors related to such things as transportation, closeness of health-care support, and costs.

Manifestations. Failure of support systems is reflected in a variety of signs and symptoms. There is a higher-than-normal divorce rate among end-stage renal disease patients. One sees teenagers failing to accept the limitations of the regular schedule of dialysis-treatment regimen—the appointments, the diet, and the medications, often because of peer pressure. Some patients become socially isolated from their home, friends, and family because of having to live closer to a dialysis-treatment center. Patients report that some family members or friends are afraid of becoming involved with chronically ill persons—their needs are too great and it creates guilt feelings. The nurse may see the physical signs and symptoms associated with noncompliance with regimen, or notice depression even to the point of loss of will to live, or the will to continue such a limited existence.

Attitude Toward Time

Failure of one of the body's life-sustaining systems is obviously a threat to one's future. This is true even when the state of the art in treatment offers promise via dialysis and kidney transplant. The status of the person's will to live, to plan for a future, is a strength or a risk that influences his participation in both the biomedical treatment and the management of daily living.

Risk Factors.   Factors that influence the attitude toward time (the present and future orientation includes the unknown and uncertain outcome of end-stage renal disease), the dependence upon the "machine" and those who run it for life, and the transplant status are major influences. Cultural and religious beliefs and/or life philosophies tend to shape the time orientation. The stage of the disease also tends to be a variable (e.g. pre-diagnosis, less than one year, or more than one year). The presence of other diseases that complicate the health picture may add to the risk of seeing no future. Use of denial as a coping mechanism also may prevent a person from planning realistically for the future.

Manifestations.   Attitude toward time can be noted in several ways. The nurse may see a patient who can make no decisions related to his own death. That is, he makes no will; he never talks about what if things do not go as hoped. Other patients dwell on the past, making no plans for the future; they look forward to nothing. Some work at living one day at a time, trying to make the most of each day, yet not looking forward to the weeks or months ahead. On the other hand, one sees those who are aggressively planning a lifestyle that includes the problems of end-stage renal disease and its treatments.

Recognition of Change in Body
Response to Activities in Daily Living

Much of the capacity to adapt one's lifestyle to the regimen required to live with end-stage renal disease is associated with the patient's ability to relate body response to activities of daily living. If there is a failure to recognize how one's patterns and activities in daily living alter the body response, there is risk that patients will not be as perceptive and sensitive in making appropriate modifications. On the other hand, there are risks if the patient becomes totally preoccupied with body response to the exclusion of all other aspects of living.

Risk Factors.   The level of denial of the disease will at times enable the patient to dissociate his activities of daily living with changes in his physical condition. At times the desire to engage in particular activities may also cause the patient to deny a relationship between them and body response. In the reverse situation, chronic illness leaves the person feeling "sub-par" most of the time and any one who has previously given neurotic attention to physical symptoms in the past is likely to give undue significance to minor body changes and to construct non-valid relationships between activities of daily living and body response.

Manifestations.   When the patient is insensitive to body response, the nurse will see a denial of presenting symptoms and signs even at times when there is visible evidence of change. The reverse situation will be evidenced by the patient's calling or reporting minor symptoms and attaching great significance to each one—a cold is seen as bronchial pneumonia.

Mobility—Attitudes
Toward Restrictions in Travel

Patients whose renal disease is treated by dialysis experience real restrictions in the amount of time they may be away from "the machine." While there are a growing number of commercial dialysis clinics throughout the country where a patient may make appointments for dialysis in other states, it is not without some problems and hazards. Thus there are *lifelong* limitations, or at least difficulties in traveling out of range of one's usual dialysis setting. This can create emotional as well as lifestyle complications, which will be important for the nurse to consider.

Risk Factors.   Factors that influence mobility include money, Hepatitis Australian Antigen (HAA) status, frequency of dialysis, age, and past lifestyle. If a patient is HAA-positive, most dialysis facilities will refuse to treat them secondary to the chance of contamination of that unit. Beyond this is the willingness of the individual to take risks and to exert both skill and assertiveness in organizing the health-care system to meet the needs associated with gaining effective, individualized dialysis outside the usual setting. Satisfaction with limited mobility may be related to past traveling lifestyle. For example a person who has traveled extensively either through his work or social activities may find it more difficult to remain in one locale than a person who has not traveled so much. One other factor is strongly influential. That is the availability of dialysis services in geographic areas to which the individual wishes to travel.

Manifestations.   A positive HAA status that prevents dialysis in other locations alerts the nurse to consider mobility a high-risk problem. Patients may make statements indicating a fear of traveling because of a lack of confidence in treatment in unfamiliar settings. Restricted financial resources can also indicate that travel will be restricted and can alert the nurse to consider patient-family response in terms of their usual or preferred mobility.

Grooming and Body Image

Usual patterns of grooming and the patient's body image are jeopardized in end-stage renal disease being treated by dialysis. This too is an area the nurse thinks of when sorting out associated problems of daily living.

Risk Factors.   Conditions that alert the nurse to consider daily living problems associated with body image and grooming include: extreme weight fluctuations that alter the clothing one can wear as well as one's appearance, the presence of a fistula or cannula as well as associated scarring from previous openings, anemia that creates a sallow pale appearance as well as fatigue, which diminishes the energy for grooming, and the age of the patient, which could influence the sense of importance of appearance.

Manifestations.   Certain signs cue the nurse to consider diagnoses associated with body image. These include the thinning of hair in women, sallowness of complexion secondary to anemia, scarring of arms and legs from numerous vascular surgeries, and extremely large veins in the arm from fistulae. The nurse may also see changes in grooming patterns—less care being taken, or depression and comments that indicate the person feels unattractive.

Level and Strategies of Denial

In a chronic disease in which alterations in patterns of daily living are a major factor in managing to stabilize one's health status, long-term denial is a particularly hazardous defense mechanism. This is a problem area to which the renal nurse is alert.

Risk Factors.   Two groups of patients seem to use denial as a defense mechanism for a longer period than do other groups. The first group are middle-aged males with many home, family, and work responsibilities. In the second high-risk group are individuals who have a strong need to belong and not to be different from others in their social groups.

Manifestations.   Several cues suggest that the nurse should consider *denial* as the basis for problems in managing daily living with end-stage renal disease being treated with dialysis. Noncompliance with the dietary regimen and the associated weight changes is a frequent sign. When the patient is on home dialysis one may see an irregularity in the scheduling of their dialyzing sessions. Those who are being dialyzed in a clinic setting may show a pattern of lateness for their appointments and more than the usual maneuvering to alter the number of dialyzing treatments to a lower number per week.

Restricted Ability to Learn New Procedures and Alterations in Lifestyle

Some individuals are less able to learn the skills and knowledge that must be assimilated in order to live with end-stage renal disease and dialysis. This inability to learn compromises their effectiveness in managing their pathophysiology and daily living.

Risk Factors.   Basic intelligence is one factor—some individuals have the capacity to learn more readily than others do. However, a high level of intelligence is not an automatic assurance of effectiveness in learning the skills and routines of living with end-stage renal disease. It has been noted that some highly intelligent patients also have the capacity to consider more of the options, more variables, more risks, and more problems. For those without this capacity, the learning is not complicated by as many considerations. Persons with a high degree of common sense and practicality seem to fare the best in adjusting to the new skills and knowledge to be assimilated.

Concurrent diseases and their biomedical management can also alter the person's capacity and stamina for learning. Often the resulting weakness and manifestations affect both the desire and ability to engage in learning. Common concurrent diseases that complicate the person's learning include diabetes and cardiac and respiratory disease.

Manifestations.   The nurse activates diagnoses in the area of *restricted learning in the face of several cues.* They tend to become obvious early and persist. In early contacts, the nurse will notice that patients either do not ask questions or ask the same questions repeatedly as if they have never been answered. When the nurse begins either to teach or to test previously taught material, that patient often changes the subject. When a topic is discussed a second or third time, the patient behaves as if he has never heard of it before. These patients are expected to monitor their weight, yet in clinic they will ask clinic personnel to weigh them because they can't learn how to use the scale. They do not learn how to take their own blood pressure. One hears, "I just can't learn how to do that—it's too complicated. These are the patients who don't take responsibility even for washing their fistula with phisohex or betadyne. Over time they tend not to gain independence, nor do they show initiative in managing their lives.

Summary

The ten categories of data that have been discussed form the critical elements for consideration in the renal nurses' diagnostic reasoning. These are high-risk problem areas to which they are alert. Patients have problems in these areas frequently, and failure to diagnose and help patients to manage problems in these areas significantly affects their well-being. It is logical then to predict that many of the diagnostic hypotheses are likely to be generated from this pool of possibilities.

ACTIVATION OF DIAGNOSTIC HYPOTHESES AND HYPOTHESIS TESTING

End-stage renal disease being treated with dialysis on an ongoing basis gives nurses regular opportunities every few days to encounter the patient and enlarge or refine the data base. Thus the pace of activation and refinement of diagnostic hypotheses may take a more gradual pace than it does in other nursing settings where these conditions do not prevail. However, because the maintenance of relative well-being in this disease is so dependent upon lifestyle in conjunction with medical therapy, the accuracy of nursing diagnosis and the effectiveness of nursing treatment strategies in assisting the patient to manage his daily living are crucial.

Diagnostic reasoning in this clinical specialty tends to take on the same pattern as that frequently encountered in other clinical areas. That is, the first cluster of cues most often results in activation of a rather general diagnostic category. This preliminary diagnostic hypothesizing enables the clinician to retrieve more specific diagnostic categories that are generally associated with the identified problem area. And, along with the potential specific diagnostic areas, the clinical retrieves the areas of inquiry that will enable a decision to confirm, refine or rule out each of the diagnostic possibilities being considered.

An example may illustrate this. The nurse sees in the patient's data field one or more or the following cues:

> extreme fluid weight gains between dialysis; complaints
>   that clothing and shoes don't fit,
> complaints of thirst and/or "bloating,"
> persistent high-serum-potassium values,
> low-serum proteins,
> loss of appetite for meat,
> preoccupation with food and drink,
> complaints of orthopnea, and
> complaints of social isolation secondary to dietary
>   restrictions.

Such cues in the data field are likely to cause the clinician to activate the general diagnostic category of *difficulty in living with dietary restrictions.*

This diagnosis of the existence of a problem is an initial level of diagnostic reasoning. However such a general diagnosis lacks the specificity needed to prescribe definitive treatment.

From the diagnosis of the general problem—*difficulty with the dietary regimen*—several more specific problem areas may be retrieved, along with areas of inquiry needed to determine whether any one or more of these problem areas exist for the patient. These diagnostic possibilities could include the following:

Home/family environment deterring dietary management

☐ Is the home environment a major factor in the
  ineffective dietary management this patient is
  engaged in?

- [ ] Who is doing the shopping and cooking?
- [ ] How many people are eating together with the patient?
- [ ] What are the usual food/salting/fluid patterns for the group that eats together and the one who does the shopping and cooking?
- [ ] What family, cultural, and interpersonal influences are shaping the patient's dietary behavior?

Social/work life and the dietary regimen

- [ ] What social/employment activities or patterns affect the patient's diet and eating patterns?

Other diseases that modify the patient's dietary management

- [ ] Are there symptoms of the other diseases that are modifying the patient's capacity to participate in this dietary regimen?
- [ ] Are dietary-fluid regimens prescribed for treatment of other diseases incongruent with the renal diet? What are the areas of incongruence?

Personal preferences, motivation, and learning ability that influence participation in the dietary regimen

- [ ] To what extent do the patient's preferences and previous dietary patterns create difficulties in adhering to the present diet?
- [ ] To what extent is the patient's stage in the denial–acceptance sequence of adaptation to the disease and treatment affecting his participation in dietary control?
- [ ] Is the patient's knowledge about food, and/or his ability to learn about his diet and his disease, a factor in his management of nutrition in daily living?
- [ ] How much influence can the factor of body image (weight fluctuation and its effect on dress, appearance, grooming) have on motivation to participate effectively in the dietary regimen?

The gathering of data in these areas should permit the diagnostician to make a much more specific formulation of the patient's presenting problem, one which will be more useful in planning for treatment. In a hypothetical example, the nurse might discover that the family is the major factor in dietary compliance. (The patient is eating with four other family members where high-sodium foods and salt consumption are the norm, and alterations are not well tolerated by the family or food preparer. The patient shares these preferences and also has a strong need not to be "different." This has in turn prolonged his use of denial as a defense mechanism.) The nurse could have ruled out the lack of the patient's ability to learn, but ruled in a problem with the food preparer's ability or desire to learn. Concurrent diseases, work, and non-family social activities would be ruled out as factors of the problem. In this hypothetical case then, the nutrition problems could be narrowed down to one multi-faceted problem: the patient in his home environment, previous home food patterns, and his relationships with the food preparer as well as other members of the family. Such a delimitation of the diagnosis enables the focus and strategies of treatment to emerge. It also suggests the logical prognostic variables in the problem as well as potential evidence of response to management.

Differential diagnosis also becomes important in terms of the focus of treatment. It can be seen, from the major categories of problem areas associated with living with end-stage renal disease, that there is a great deal of interrelatedness. It becomes important to determine which problems are the geneses of other problems. For example, fatigue, secondary to a low hematocrit, may contribute significantly to the capacity and desire of the patient to work on managing the diet and fluid restrictions in daily living. Or, the reverse might be true that the failure to manage the diet is a major factor in increasing the patient's fatigue level. In both instances, energy levels and the managing of dietary restrictions are elements, but the diagnosis will be structured differently—the perspective will be different.

Just as a valid, adequate, well-organized data base is the foundation for a precise and accurate diagnosis, so the diagnosis and associated knowledge of its underlying mechanisms becomes the structure upon which the treatment decisions are based. For example, if the low hematocrit is causing fatigue that is likely to be a problem for x number of weeks until the body has adjusted, then support systems to assist the patient in managing would be appropriate; and the pace, timing, and level of teaching–learning expectations would need to be geared to energy levels on a week-by-week basis. If, on the other hand, the organic basis for fatigue is ruled out and dietary mismanagement is confirmed by data, the treatment plan and motivation may well be directed toward helping the patient 1) to see the link between diet and energy levels and 2) to find acceptable strategies for living in a reasonably satisfying way with the food and fluid regimen.

SUMMARY

Diagnostic categories in nursing patients with end-stage renal disease share many similarities to those of terminal cancer patients, as described in Chapter 5. Important differences are apparent as well. The end-stage renal dialysis patient is undergoing therapy, with the hope of maintaining a quality of living, rather than dying. Consequently, much of his effort is directed toward activities involved in a treatment regimen, like in the case of a person with diabetes. These empirically derived categories of diagnosis are steps toward development of a classification of nursing diagnoses common to persons with chronic illness requiring life-long complex treatment regimens.

CHAPTER SEVEN

Diagnostic Reasoning in Nursing Care of Persons with Diabetes Mellitus

Carol G. Blainey

A good deal of the responsibility that professional nurses have in working with people who have chronic disease conditions lies in the area of developing the person's ability to manage his or her own condition on a day-to-day basis. Contact with health professionals is infrequent and brief, as compared to the all-day-every-day management responsibility carried by people who have chronic disease. Coping with changed and changing statuses in activities of daily living is another dimension of the situation in chronic illness. These two components, management of treatment regimens and coping with changed and changing statuses in ADL, are inextricably linked. Difficulty in coping with changed status may interfere with the person's ability to carry out prescribed management regimens and failure to comply with treatment regimens may increase problems in coping in ADL.

Contents of this chapter will deal with diagnostic reasoning as it pertains to coping status in the activities of daily living. Sexual functioning is used as the illustration. Diabetes is the prototype condition as an example of—

- a condition requiring constant surveillance and management by affected individuals, and
- a condition with potentially profound effects on activities of daily living.

PRE-ENTRY FACTORS

Nursing Specialty

The specialized area of nursing people with diabetes influences the areas evaluated with respect to activities of daily living (ADL) and

149

demands of daily living (DDL). Sexual function and intimacy are among the many areas of daily living affected by the disease, diabetes. Recognition by the nurse of the potential for problems of intimacy is a function of experience gained in working with persons with diabetes, and is indicative of the value that the nurse specialist places on acknowledging and allowing client expression of sexuality.

From the outset of this discussion, it is recognized that sexual functioning has a large psychogenic component complicating the situation. One's religious beliefs, social mores, and previous experience are involved in this psychogenic component. In addition, there is not a long past history of open discussion regarding sexual expression in general or between people and health professionals. These complexities militate against health professionals making a conscious consideration of coping status in the area of sexuality. There can be a feeling of awkwardness on the part of the health professional due to lack of experience in dealing with sexuality as well as lack of existing knowledge regarding precision in determining causes or treatment of problems.

Sexuality has been selected as an illustration of this diagnostic process because it is an important concern to most people and because it increases the risk of difficulty-in-coping for people with diabetes.

Pre-existing Patient Data

The data base pertinent to activating the hypothesis "actual or potential sexual dysfunction" includes the health history, physical examination, laboratory data, and previous progress records, all of which provide information regarding the individual's current status and the development of the disease process. Specific data necessary would be laboratory studies that rule out medically correctable endocrine dysfunction as a basis for sexual dysfunction.

ENTRY TO THE DATA FIELD

The typical first meeting with the client is in an outpatient clinic. The person may be newly diagnosed or may have had a diagnosis of *diabetes* for some years. To begin, the current physiological status of their condition is established.

Following is a framework of pivotal questions one might pose to detect difficulties in coping with ADL in relation to diabetes mellitus:

☐ How has having diabetes affected your body?

- ☐ How do you feel having diabetes will affect your body over time?
- ☐ What do you believe caused your diabetes?
- ☐ How do you feel having diabetes has or will affect your life?
- ☐ What do you believe you can do to minimize the effects of having diabetes?
- ☐ Where does treating diabetes rank in your current personal priority list?

Responses to these questions provide opportunities to verbalize current problems and concerns for the future. Validating the person's intellectual understanding and psychomotor abilities to implement his or her management regimen adds information and provides an opportunity to develop a relationship of mutual respect and to affirm the nurse's genuine concern and credibility. Once this relationship has been established and the basic ability to carry out the treatment plan is established one can move to the question of the individual's status at coping with sexuality in the face of the condition and the treatment regimen. The professional nurse's manner of conveying comfort and a recognition of an acceptance of sexuality work to increase people's willingness and ability to discuss their concerns. To help focus the individual who is vague or global in his responses to the pivotal questions one can use sensitive clarification techniques or, possibly, offer the option of talking to someone else, perhaps someone of the same sex. Cues to difficulties in sexual functioning are sometimes vague and difficult to interpret. Interest or lack of interest in sexual activity by the individual's partner undoubtedly influences his or her own feeling.

Activation of Diagnostic Hypothesis: Actual or Potential Sexual Dysfunction

Nursing diagnoses commonly occurring in the area of sexuality in people who have diabetes are:

lack of information regarding potential sexual dysfunction,

unresolved concerns regarding potential difficulties with sexual expression, satisfaction, and reproduction, and

depression regarding impotence or lack of satisfaction from sexual expression.

The following comments illustrate the diagnostic thinking process utilized in arriving at these diagnoses.

A number of factors in the recorded history and initial interview with the client suggest high potential for sexual dysfunction. These include sex, age, duration of diabetes, diabetic control, and presence of end-organ disease. Once these cues to the potential diagnosis are present, data regarding the individual's priority systems and support systems serve to validate the probability of that diagnosis for a given individual.

Sex.   Men seem more likely to be threatened by a disruption in sexual functioning by virtue of the visibility of sexual arousal and hence other's awareness of potency. The psychogenic component of sexual function is strong but unmeasurable. To be specific, fear of inability to achieve erection can interfere with the ability to do so. Interacting with this psychogenic element is the fact that 50% of men over 30 years-of-age who have diabetes have diabetes-based sexual impotence (Ellenberg, 1979, p. 4; Schiavi, 1979, p. 10). The physiological bases of the sexual impotence are rooted in damage to the vascular and neurological systems. Sperm count and motility are decreased, and the incidence of retrograde ejaculation is increased in men who have diabetes.

Women who have diabetes have decreased fertility and increased incidence of incomplete pregnancies as well as increased incidence of problems in their newborn babies. Oral birth control pills as a means of contraception frequently cause difficulties in control of blood glucose. Urinary tract and vaginal infections are frequent in women with poorly controlled diabetes. In addition, there is considerable anecdotal, and some documented, evidence that satisfaction from sexual intercourse is compromised in women who have diabetes.

The increased incidence of diabetes in offspring of people who have diabetes, together with a decreased life expectancy, give rise to questions of whether to have one's natural children. Moreover, people who develop diabetes in their middle and later years may have concerns about whether they would have had their own children had they known they would develop diabetes in their later years.

Age.   Young men who are impotent or fear impotence can present as depressed or aggressive and angry. As mentioned earlier, these men may also be concerned about whether they should reproduce. Middle-aged men may sense a general decline in all areas of functioning, and presence or fear of impotence may be adding to other problems. Older men may feel awkward because they believe they should not be, but in fact are, concerned about sexual functioning.

Young women are concerned about reliable and acceptable birth control methods that are appropriate for women with diabetes. Their dilemma of whether or not they should have their natural children is coupled with the double-edged problem of increased difficulties in controlling their own diabetes and increased potential for problems of the fetus and newborn.

Young, middle, and advanced-aged women who have diabetes have an increased incidence of vaginal and urinary tract infections, which interfere with satisfactory sexual functioning. In addition there is the not-completely-confirmed data showing a general decrease in satisfaction from sexual intercourse among women with diabetes that is not related to infectious processes of the genitourinary system.

Duration of Diagnosis of Diabetes.   Length of time of presence of diabetes has an impact on sexual function in that longer duration is generally associated with more male impotence. Infrequently, impotence is the presenting symptom of the individual with undiagnosed diabetes. There is no firm data on how time affects sexual functioning in women. As time progresses, there is generally more damage to vascular and nervous systems in people who have diabetes. There is some evidence that people who are recently diagnosed tend to be more concerned with following therapeutic regimens, and as time goes on, they tend to become more casual in compliance.

Ease of Control.   It is generally believed that keeping the blood glucose at more normal levels may improve sexual functioning. Certainly, the effect that careful control would have on minimizing urinary and vaginal infections would improve sexual function. The threat or event of spontaneous hypoglycemia with exercise may interfere with sexual activity.

Amount of End-Organ Disease.   The presence of more damage to vascular and nervous systems, which is not always related to duration of the condition, usually results in more male sexual impotence. Drugs necessary to control blood pressure may interfere with sexual potency. The devastating effects of blindness and renal failure threaten usual patterns of sexual expression.

Body Weight.   Many people with non-insulin-dependent diabetes mellitus are obese and they may have a negative body image, which can include feeling sexually undesirable.

Priorities System.   The rank of sexual expression in the priority systems of individuals and their significant others influences the impact of change or threats to change in sexuality. Further, the value an individual places on treating his diabetes may influence sexual functioning. For example, if family and work are taking precedence over sexual expression, a person may not carefully follow regimens and may be symptomatic (*i.e.*, suffer from fatigue or vaginal infections). This can lead to interference with sexual functioning.

Support Systems.   Interpersonal support systems clearly influence sexuality. Having significant others who are willing to work with problems improves the outlook of coping with changing sexual functioning. As mentioned earlier, there is a strong psychogenic component in sexual function and if people feel supported, the psychogenic component is more likely to be positive.

An individual's economic status and health insurance coverage may impact sexual functioning in that lack of funds or insurance coverage may preclude some forms of treatment, such as penile implants or psychological counseling.

Summary

The list below summarizes the risk potential in people who have diabetes mellitus.

Summary of Risk Potential for Sexual Dysfunction in People Who Have Diabetes

At high risk for difficulty-in-coping status in area of sexuality

impotence	taking medications that may cause impotence, high alcohol intake
male	
young	
considerable end-organ disease	long standing diagnosis of diabetes
high priority of sexuality	
low economic status	frequent urinary tract infections and vaginal infections
strong desire for own children	
primarily external sense of locus of control	difficulty with control of blood glucose
	minimal support systems

At less risk for difficulties in coping status in area of sexuality

female	smooth control of blood glucose
middle-aged	low priority of sexuality
advanced-aged	high-economic status
recent diagnosis of diabetes	strong support systems
not taking any drugs other than insulin	no desire for children
strong internal locus of control	

Consideration of these areas provides input to rule in or out the previously noted nursing diagnosis:

- ☐ Lack of information regarding potential sexual dysfunction.
- ☐ Unresolved concerns regarding potential difficulties with sexual expression, satisfaction, and reproduction.
- ☐ Depression regarding impotence or lack of satisfaction from sexual expression.

HYPOTHESIS TESTING

Differentiating Among Nursing Diagnoses

First a *general* diagnosis is made: *dysfunction in coping with regards to sexuality*. This is followed by the process of differentiating that general diagnosis into more specific components. The following consideration of risk factors raises the possibility of the existence of the diagnosis—*lack of information regarding potential sexual dysfunction:*

adolescence or young adult

female or male

brief duration of diagnosis of diabetes

high priority of sexuality

strong desire for natural children, and

requirement for medications that have the side effect of impotence.

Risk factors associated with the diagnosis of *unresolved concerns regarding potential difficulties with sexual expression and reproduction* are:

any age

both sexes

any duration of diagnosis

high priority of sexuality

evidence of end-organ disease

frequent UTI

recurrent vaginal infections

strong desire for natural children

minimal support systems

external locus of control, and

low socio-economic status

The diagnosis of *depression regarding impotence or lack of satisfaction from sexual activity* is attended by this collection of risk factors:

☐ any age, male or female, impotence
☐ high priority of sexuality
☐ minimal support systems
☐ external locus of control
☐ difficulty with control of blood glucose
☐ frequent UTI and vaginal infection
☐ low socio-economic status.

Prognosis

The prognosis of *successful coping with difficulties in sexuality* is directly related to the number of risk factors present. In addition, the coping status is not static. Some times will be better than others depending on the changeable nature of the risk factors.

Treatment

Recognizing and openly discussing the difficulties of coping with problems of sexuality seem to reduce much of the accumulated pressure around the problem. Validating people's correct understanding of factors of inheritance, pregnancy with diabetes, and potential for impotence in men is a part of treatment when the diagnosis is *lack of understanding.* When the diagnosis is *unresolved concerns regarding potential difficulties with sexual expression and reproduction,* treatment includes validation of appropriate knowledge and techniques to aid the individual in clarifying the specific basis of his or her concerns.

When the diagnosis is *depression from sexual impotence,* validating understanding of the physician's explanation of medical diagnostic processes and various forms of surgical intervention is an important part of nursing therapy.

Encouraging open discussion between the affected individual and professional nurse, and affected individual and significant others, is a crucial component of care. The person with diabetes can be given suggestions for opening sentences to begin discussion with a significant other. Consideration of psychological intimacy and forms of physical closeness that do not require coitus can serve to put the specific act in clearer perspective.

Once the problem has been discussed and an open relationship between health professional and patient is established, the person can dictate the frequency with which he or she chooses to address the concern. Clearly, some individuals will require referral to specialists in person and sexual counseling.

Self-management of any chronic condition is facilitated by contact with the same health professional. This obvious statement is even more crucial in the case of diabetes and, more specifically, in the case of difficulty in coping with changed or potentially changed sexuality. Careful documentation of the nursing process can serve as a second-best situation if the person cannot routinely see the same professional nurse.

SUMMARY

Sexuality is but one area of daily living affected by a chronic disorder such as diabetes. This chapter has described the thinking process by which knowledge of the physiologic effects of the disease, risk factors, associated disease, patient characteristics, and the value system of the patient all interact to produce a differential nursing diagnosis within a general category—*actual or potential sexual problem.*

BIBLIOGRAPHY

Symposium on Sex and Diabetes. Diabetes Care. 2(1):1–31, January/February 1979

Ellenberg M: Impotence in Diabetes The Neurologic Factor. Ann Intern Med 75:213–219, 1971

Ellenberg M: Sexual aspects of the female diabetic. Mt Sinai J Med 44:495, 1977

Ellenberg M: Sex and Diabetes: A Comparison Between Men and Women Diabetes Care 2:4–8 Jan/Feb 1979

Kolodny RC: Sexual Dysfunction in Diabetic Females. Diabetes 20:557, 1971

Rubin A and Babbott D: Impotence and diabetes mellitus. JAMA 168:498–500, 1958

Schiavi RC and Hogan B: Psychological Aspects of Sexual Problems. Diabetes Care 2:9–17, January/February 1979

Schoffling K et al: Disorders of Sexual Function in Male Diabetics. Diabetes 12:519–527, 1963

Unsain I and Goodwin M: Effects on Sexual Function. In Nursing Management of Diabetes Mellitus, 2nd Edition, St. Louis: C.V. Mosby, 1982

CHAPTER EIGHT

Diagnostic Reasoning in a Critical Care Setting

Pamela H. Mitchell

Although the setting in which diagnostic decision-making takes place is an acknowledged factor influencing the mental processing of data, the available literature presumes that the encounter between health practitioner and patient (or client) occurs in a stable setting.

Textbooks that teach history-taking and analysis of a symptom generally approach both from the setting in which practitioner and patient actively exchange information and in which the patient is presumed to be physiologically stable. Further, those nursing textbooks that use this approach tend to be intended for the "expanded role"—the nurse who combines medical and nursing diagnostic decision-making. Thus, the "analysis of a symptom" material is directed toward the detection of disease and pathology. Some such textbooks do include material regarding the approach to the comatose patient, or to the patient in physiologically unstable condition (as in the emergency room, following trauma).

Furthermore, all examples used in research regarding diagnostic decision-making presume that the patient can supply a coherent history and respond to data-seeking inquiries of the diagnostician. Many of the studies regarding diagnostic thinking in nursing do not presuppose an alert, stable patient, but rather start from a symptom or sign and ask the study respondents to determine the likely cause of that symptom (Gordon, 1980; Aspinall, 1976). Further, the few studies that have been conducted regarding nursing decision-making processes focus on decision-making in the realm of action or management (Grier, 1976; Hansen and Thomas, 1968).

In settings such as critical-care units, patients are, by definition, in highly unstable or potentially unstable states. Consequently, in such settings, the patterns of data-generation and hypothesis-formation that are initiated by the patient's chief concern are not the pri-

159

mary sources of information-processing in the initial encounter, and generally in subsequent encounters. Rather the nurse's diagnostic approach to the patient is shaped by two equally important, and often competing factors: 1) the stability of psychophysiological functioning (is the patient better or worse?) and 2) the extent to which normal routines of daily living (including life support functions) must be supplemented by nursing care. Because the patient's state can and may change rapidly, every encounter is focused toward determining the state of these two dimensions, with subsequent management of resources subject to continual revision. Stability of physiologic function may be considered a shared nursing and medical focus.

The more purely nursing diagnostic perspective concerns itself with linking the data on status of internal resources (physiological-psychological stability and levels of capability) to the presenting activities and demands of daily living in the ICU.

To exemplify the process in a more concrete manner, this chapter will examine the processes in relation to persons with life-threatening neurological disease. It is not essential that the reader be familiar with neurological nursing to understand the thinking processes.

PRE-ENCOUNTER INFLUENCES

In these acute and critical-care settings, the priorities of data collection, the focus of data collection, and the form in which the data are available are all strongly influenced by the dynamic and highly technological nature of the setting. They are further shaped by the priority given in that setting to maintenance of biologic life. The "givens," or the factors that shape one's focus of data collection even prior to the first encounter with the patient, all relate to the instability of physiologic function. The factors include the setting, with its emphasis on involvement of multiple physiologic systems, the complex technology of the setting, and the practitioner's area of specialty knowledge.

Nursing Specialty

The specialized nursing focus of the practitioner is an important pre-encounter influence upon entry to the diagnostic search. Unless the practitioner remains open to the interrelationship of the multiple body systems affected, such focus can serve to constrict the data field prematurely. I use three categories of information regarding patient status that serve to remind me to consider factors outside my specialty focus, and to remind me of the nursing focus. Those categories are 1) general state of the patient, 2) nervous system state, and 3) self-care state; in that order of evaluation. In terms of the critical-care setting, the *general status* includes the A, B, C's: airway, breathing, circulation. *Nervous system status* includes: consciousness, mentation, movement, sensation, and integrated regulation. (Mitchell et al, 1984). *Self care state* includes: bathing, toileting, moving, feeding, communicating, socializing, and assuming role activities (Benoliel, McCorkle, and Young, 1980). Decisions regarding abilities in self-care are based on the findings of general status, nervous system status and the medical management regimen.

The categories are the same ones I use in a chronic-care setting, but the rapidity of data collection, the kinds of data used and the active involvement of the patient vary with the setting.

Setting

The setting is a highly visible influence on the diagnostic areas the clinician attends to, and the kind of data available. By definition, most patients in critical-care units are potentially or actually physiologically unstable and highly vulnerable to changes in their environment. The preeminent concern of all those in the setting—indeed its *raison d'être*—is whether the patient has become more unstable. The goal of all therapies is to restore stability so that healing may take place.

Multisystem Involvement. A factor in the setting is the complexity of the pathological process in most of the patients. Because the regulation of physiologic systems is highly integrated, major breakdown of any one system ultimately affects all. This is certainly the case in many severe neurologic disorders, for the nervous system is the ultimate integrator of all others. Multiple trauma is another example of the multisystem involvement. Even in the supposedly "single system" units such as coronary-care units, failure of the heart results in secondary failure of lungs, kidney, and brain. Consequently, nursing and medical diagnosis in these settings cannot focus exclusively on the one system known best to the practitioner.

Complex Technology. Complex technology is another important influence on the clinician's approach to data gathering and information processing in this setting. While technology influences any setting, it is most highly visible in the modern intensive-care unit. Thus, all health professionals in these settings not only gather data from the machines and computers, but must interpret the data in terms of its meaning: patient malfunction or machine malfunction. The technology does not replace the human observer; it refines and sharpens observations and adds to our ability to evaluate the internal environment of the patient. Technological equipment is generally viewed as assisting in the evaluation of the patient's medical status—that is, the function of diseased organs and organ systems. Nurses who use that data tend to use it from the medical frame of reference. As will be demonstrated later in the chapter, these data can be used equally well to test nursing diagnostic hypotheses, and to evaluate the effect of nursing care regimens.

Nursing Focus in the Setting.   A final factor that influences diagnosis is the focus of nursing care in this setting. The intensity of nursing observation was certainly a major impetus for the development of special-care units. However, in the last analysis, patients are in these units because they need *intensive nursing care, meaning that they require maximal supplementation of their own disrupted internal resources to accomplish activities and demands of daily living.* In many cases this includes even the most elemental aspects of breathing, feeding, moving, and communicating. Consequently, crucial nursing decision-making is focused on determining the amount and kind of supplemental care needs. In Orem's framework, diagnoses lead to the design of a wholly compensatory care system. (Orem 1980)

ENTRY AND PATTERNS
OF EARLY DATA SEARCH

The initial encounter with the patient may begin with a telephone report of a patient to be admitted, at change-of-shift report because one is assigned to care for the patient, or during a verbal or written consultation regarding some aspect of that patient's care or status. Consequently, one has a "set" regarding stability or instability.

The setting and the specialty focus also serve to "set" and limit the potential diagnostic hypotheses generated in the initial encounter. Medical and nursing responsibilities and diagnoses overlap to a greater degree than in other settings. Because of this phenomenon, greater space is devoted in this chapter than in other chapters to nursing diagnostic thinking in this shared area.

ACTIVATION OF
DIAGNOSTIC HYPOTHESES

Diagnostic reasoning in the shared nursing/medical area is focused on the general area of *physiologic stability as it poses a threat to life.* The more purely nursing diagnostic area can be categorized broadly as that which determines the extent and kind of *imbalance between internal resources and activities/demands of daily living*. The data gathered and conclusions reached with regard to the shared biomedical diagnostic area (life-threatening physiologic stability) cannot be readily separated from the reasoning processes necessary for determining the nature of deficits and dysfunction requiring self-care supplementation. Therefore, the following sections are arranged to demonstrate the flow of thinking process from one area to the other. The list below illustrates major categories of nursing diagnoses in the area of neurocritical care.

Common Diagnostic Areas in Neurocritical Care

Major category: Depleted Resources Relative to Demands
   of Daily Living
     Risk to Psychophysiologic Integrity
       Immobility
          Physical, Social, Psychological
          Subunits: Risk for skin breakdown, muscle
               disuse, atrophy,
               thrombophlebitis, constipation,
               urinary retention
       Sensory deprivation syndrome
       Impaired verbal communication
       Nutritional deficit secondary to impaired oral
         feeding
       Impaired responsiveness
       Depersonalization
       Sleep Deprivation
     Diminished Adaptive Reserves
       Contributing pathophysiologic state
         Ventilatory insufficiency
         Respiratory insufficiency
         Circulatory insufficiency—decreased cardiac
                output
               decreased
                 peripheral
                 resistance
               decreased venous
                 return

(*continued on next page*)

Increased intracranial pressure

Decreased or absent autonomic regulatory reflexes (*e.g.*, spinal shock)

Hypermetabolic state

Diminished Capacity for Self-Care (ADL)

Impaired responsiveness

Paralysis

Diminished adaptive reserve

Pain

Physiological Stability as Related to Threat to Life

The stability of physiological systems is evaluated in order of the *hierarchy* regarding threat to life. Therefore, airway, breathing, and circulation are evaluated before evaluation of nervous system functioning. In actuality, it is often difficult to tell when an experienced practitioner ends one evaluation and begins another, for the observations are integrated in the mind.

General hypotheses in this area of physiological stability are a) ventilatory insufficiency and b) circulatory insufficiency. The specific diagnoses that describe the nature and extent of life-threatening disturbances in ventilation, circulation, and cellular respiration are well described in textbooks dealing with the diagnostic areas shared between medicine and nursing and will not be repeated here. Risk factors and general manifestations of the class of diagnoses are summarized below.

Ventilatory–Respiratory Insufficiency

Risk Factors. Patients with multi-trauma, with primary pulmonary disease, and with certain neurologic disorders (described under "Neurologic Stability") are all at high risk for ventilatory and respiratory insufficiency. In addition, those who have markedly decreased mobility are at high risk for atelectasis and subsequent compromised respiration.

Manifestations. Observationally, one looks for patency of airway (natural or artificial), listens for sounds of secretions or fluid from humidifier, checks regular ventilator rhythms, observes the character of respiratory excursion, ventilator settings, skin color, and color of lips and nailbeds, listens for abnormal breath sounds by auscultation, and notes changes in mentation or anxiety. Additional data necessary to evaluate respiration and its relationship to CNS function are blood gases and response of intracranial pressure to suctioning. One is likely to make a mental note to look at such data after bedside observation and examination. Not only are such data important in primary evaluation of respiratory status, but because they influence the intracranial pressure. Increased intracranial pressure is a concomitant of many brain disorders in critical care, and its control is crucial to survival and potential long-term neuronal function. Consequently, data regarding respiratory status, ventilation, and asymmetric lung function will provide important clues to determine body positions likely to worsen or improve intracranial pressure status.

Circulatory Insufficiency

Risk Factors.   Risk factors are greatest in patients with primary cardiovascular disease and multitrauma patients with volume loss. Patients with spinal cord injury lose some peripheral cardiovascular reflex regulation, as may patients with polyneuropathy. CNS injury such as head injury and subarachnoid hemorrhage may also produce secondary cardiac damage.

Manifestations.   In general, abnormal function is manifested by changes in mentation, blood pressure, and observable skin color. Circulation is evaluated by color, blanching, and the presence or absence of visible edema. In many patients, electronic monitoring of electrocardiograph, arterial blood pressure, pulmonary wedge pressure, and cardiac output are available to add precision to the evaluation of cardiac function.

Neurologic Stability

Once general stability is established one looks for evidence of neurologic stability or instability. In reality, the experienced practitioner is doing both at the same time. However, they are separated here to avoid confusion.

The pattern and priority of data search regarding neurologic function are guided by the two major diagnostic hypothesis categories in which neurologic dysfunction is life-threatening. Neurologic disorders can threaten life when they 1) cause brain herniation and 2) cause respiratory insufficiency (Mitchell 1980). Consequently, physical examination and evaluation of adjunctive data (laboratory data, trends in vital signs, and so on) are geared toward early detection of patterns indicating these diagnostic categories: a) potential brain herniation, b) potential respiratory insufficiency.

Brain Herniation

Risk Factors.   Certain injuries and disorders place patients at high risk for brain herniation. Examples are severe head injury, with subsequent brain swelling and edema, any injury or metabolic illness that produces widespread brain edema, expanding mass lesions, such as tumors, epidural and subdural hematomas, intracerebral hemorrhage, postoperative brain edema after craniotomy, and the massive brain edema seen with near drowning, cerebral hypoxia, and Reye's syndrome*. Increased intracranial pressure in itself does not produce brain herniation, but is so commonly associated with entities that do, that the presence of intracranial hypertension is an important clue that brain herniation may be possible.

Brain disorders that do not create brain shift or massive swelling do not activate the diagnosis: *potential herniation*. Examples of these disorders include senile dementia of the Alzheimer type, multiple sclerosis, and epilepsy.

Manifestations.   Changes in level of consciousness, in symmetry of motor function and reflexes, and in patterns of respiration, extraocular movements, and pupillary reactions constitute the constellation of signs of brain herniation. Changes in vital signs occur so late in the process that they confirm rather than activate the hypothesis that herniation is occuring.

Ventilatory Insufficiency

Risk Factors.   Neurologically caused ventilatory insufficiency is potential in patients whose disorders affect either the brain stem areas and cranial nerves that protect the airway (the so-called "bulbar" area), or the innervation to the muscles of respiration: the diaphragm and the intercostal muscles. Disorders that affect the brain stem and its nerves include completed brain herniation, brain stem stroke, myasthenia gravis (affecting muscles innervated by the brain stem), poliomyelitis, ascending polyneuropathy (Guillian-Barre syndrome; Landry's paralysis), and diphtheric polyneuropathy. Disorders that affect the muscles of respiration include high spinal-cord injury (C2–T2; those above C4–5 affect both diaphragm and accessory muscles of respiration); amyotrophic lateral sclerosis, and muscular dystrophy. Myasthenia gravis affects muscles of swallowing, airway pro-

---

* Reye's syndrome is a disorder of children characterized by breakdown of cellular metabolic machinery. Increased intracranial pressure and liver dysfunction are the most life-threatening manifestations.

tection, and of respiration. Tetanus interferes with respiration through tetany of the muscles of respiration.

The presence of any of these medical diagnoses should activate careful evaluation of direct and laboratory data regarding respiratory status. Trends over the past few hours are more important than any single observation. Manifestations were summarized earlier in the chapter.

Psychophysiologic Stability in Relation to ADL

The popular image of critical-care nursing, and the one to which most textbook space is devoted, is that of the life-maintaining functions and the categories of diagnostic thinking just described. The majority of nursing care is, however, devoted to activities stemming from diagnoses solely within the nursing focus. These activities, such as turning, bathing, massaging, and communicating are considered such basic nursing care that many (perhaps most) critical-care nurses find it difficult to articulate the diagnoses that dictate these activities or management plans.

Common diagnostic hypotheses that relate to supplementation of daily living fall into three categories: 1) risk to psychophysiologic integrity, 2) diminished adaptive reserve capacity and 3) diminished capacity for self-care. These categories have been derived empirically from personal experience and discussions with critical-care nurses. They are consistent with common diagnoses derived from the national conference group list for cardiovascular specialists (Castles, 1982) but are organized quite differently.

The categories as a whole will be discussed briefly to give the reader an orientation to the relationship of subcategories within the overall category. Risk factors and manifestations of one diagnostic category (diminished adaptive capacity, increased intracranial pressure) will be described. Finally, the diagnostic reasoning process will be taken from symptom to management using an example from the diminished adaptive capacity, ventilatory insufficiency.

Risk to Psychophysiologic Integrity

Diagnostic hypotheses in this category are most likely to be generated by knowing the patient's medical diagnosis and/or observation of the general "state of the patient."

Activation by Medical Diagnosis. For example, the medical diagnosis: *complete spinal cord injury C5–6* immediately activates a full range of potential diagnoses in the area of risk to psychophysiological integrity. These include:

potential skin breakdown,

muscle atrophy,

grieving process,

altered elimination, and

impaired verbal communication (if a tracheostomy is
   necessary for ventilatory sufficiency).

This medical diagnosis should also generate a number of potential nursing diagnoses in the category of *diminished adaptive capacity,* to be discussed below. The activation by medical diagnosis of a set of potential nursing diagnoses is an example of cross-referencing and "chunking" by experienced diagnosticians. A novice would need to go to the patient's side and see that the patient cannot move voluntarily below the shoulders, and recall that lack of movement leads to skin breakdown. She would then note that the patient breathes shallowly (or not at all) and would recall the potential problems related to breathing and so on. The experienced neuro-nurse knows from long-term memory what functions are regulated by the C5–6 level of the spinal cord and therefore what risks to psychophysiologic integrity are posed by loss of these functions to *everyone* who has that injury. These data are stored as a unit and called forth by the term: complete injury C5–6 (*i.e.,* no physiologic transmission of impulses from central nervous system below C5–6). She then uses bedside evaluation to determine a) if there is evidence that the potential diagnoses have become actual and b) what diagnoses specific to this individual are present.

Activation by Observation of the General State of the Patient.   As described above, the novice must use this method almost exclusively, until the store of "chunk-activated" knowledge is well into memory. For all nurses, observation may prompt movement of diagnosis from the potential to actual state. For example, the presence of a tracheostomy activates the problem statement "impaired verbal communication" and a reddened coccyx activates "impending sacral decubitus" (provided one knows the manifestations of the diagnosed state).

Diminished Adaptive Reserve Capacity

Adaptation is the process of returning to equilibrium after perturbation or disruption of that steady state. Thus, adaptive reserve is that set of biological, psychological, or social resources possessed by the person, and which may be used in the process of adaptation. The critically ill person, by virtue of his or her primary disease state, is very likely to have diminished reserve capacity in one or more physiologic systems. Further, these states of diminished physiologic reserve are concomitants of the pathologic state for which the person is receiving medical therapy. Thus, much of the data used by nurse and physician in determining change or threat to life related to the primary disease process are used simultaneously by the nurse to activate hypotheses of diminished adaptive capacity.

Diagnostic hypotheses in this category are also activated by a combination of knowledge regarding a given medical diagnosis, a given pathophysiologic state (for example cardiogenic shock, intracranial hypertension) and observation of the patient.

Activation by Medical Diagnosis.   In the example used earlier, the medical diagnosis: *complete spinal cord injury at C5–6* generates a whole series of *compromised adaptive capacities:*

decreased ventilatory reserve,

loss of postural cardiovascular reflexes,

loss of peripheral temperature-regulating capacity, and

loss of urinary and bowel reflexes.

These hypotheses, when confirmed by objective data then form the basis for a nursing management plan in which challenge to the adaptive capacity of these systems is minimized by prescribed nursing treatment. For example, from the neuroanatomy portion of my knowledge packet about spinal cord injury, I know that the phrenic nerve to the diaphragm is innervated at C3–5 and that the intercostal muscles are innervated in the thoracic region. Since this person's injury is at C5–6, my knowledge of anatomy confirms the hypothesis: decreased adaptive capacity, ventilation (because the intercostal muscles are below the injury and thus receive no voluntary motor impulses). It is possible that ascending cord edema could affect phrenic nerve function as well, thus creating ventilatory insufficiency (or arrest). Vital capacity, blood gases, and other measures of pulmonary function are the objective data that will confirm or rule out inadequate ventilation. Even if basal ventilation is adequate, decreased ventilatory adaptive reserve capacity remains a diagnosis, and nursing management in the immediate phase is based on minimizing emotional upset (which requires increased ventilation) and preventing atelectasis or pneumonia (which calls on adaptive capacities). After the stage of spinal shock, pulmonary-function-test results and observations of the patients circulatory and ventilatory response to increasing activity serve as data to determine the extent or degree of reduced ventilatory adaptive capacity.

Activation by Pathophysiologic State. Some pathophysiologic states activate hypotheses of reduced adaptive capacity, regardless of the name of the disease state. For example, shock is a state occurring secondary to many diseases and which results in cellular hypoxia. Thus a patient in shock, by definition, has reduced adaptive capacity in all systems and requires a wholly compensatory nursing management plan.

Increased intracranial pressure (ICP) is another example of a pathophysiologic state that activates the hypothesis: reduced adaptive capacity. Intracranial hypertension can be present in many intracranial disorders: head injury, Reye's syndrome, tumor, massive stroke, or bleeding intracerebral aneurysm. The level of intracranial pressure alone does not sufficiently determine to what degree adaptive capacity is impaired. *At high risk* are those with increased ICP (greater than 15 mm Hg) and one or more of the following: increased amplitude of ICP waveform, high volume-pressure response (VPR) or volume-pressure index (VPI), impaired ventilation, hypercapnia, labile systemic blood pressure, and ICP pressure waves.

Reduced intracranial adaptive capacity may be *manifested* by sharp and sustained (greater than 5 min) ICP increases to environmental or positional challenge such as bedside conversations, turning, suctioning, and repositioning. Management decisions are then based on observation of the response to challenge in patients at risk and a) avoidance of activities that exceed adaptive capacity, or b) use of prescribed ICP-reducing measures prior to nursing care activities that cannot be avoided.

Activation by Observation of Patient State. Some states of reduced adaptive capacity are not obvious from medical diagnosis or pathophysiologic state. Fatigue, or increased instability of circulatory and respiratory measures are common observational cues to the decreased adaptive capacity diagnosis. Pain may also be a cue, particularly in patients with primary cardiovascular pathology. These are the cues that generate the comment "he just can't tolerate activity," which is really a diagnosis of decreased adaptive capacity.

Decreased Capacity for Self-Care

Almost by definition, critical illness implies marked decrease in the capacity for caring for one's own daily activities. Thus the setting:

critical care unit implies the general category of decreased capacity for self-care. However, determining the *extent* and *duration* of such decreased capacity is the art of critical-care nursing.

Medical diagnosis is rarely an activator of hypotheses in this category. Such terms as head injury or Guillain-Barre syndrome tell us little about the adaptive capacities and functional abilities of the person with the disease. Such a diagnosis as *complete spinal cord injury C5–6* may serve to activate diagnoses in this category because this anatomical description calls forth a knowledge packet that indicates the deficits in function for all people who are so injured. However, this part of the knowledge "chunk" is stored in terms of functions basic to self-care—responsiveness, movement, and mentation rather than pathophysiologic state. From this chunk, one knows that the person is paralyzed from shoulders down (and thus incapable of voluntary movement), has intact consciousness (if there is no accompanying head injury) has reduced adaptive capacity, particularly in ventilation, circulation, and temperature regulation, and may or may not be fully aware of the extent of his or her impairments. The logical hypothesis is complete loss of capacity for physical self-care with unknown capacity to direct- or request-preferred style of care from the caregivers.

Thus the knowledge or observation "paralysis" is one cue that activates the category of diminished self-care capacity. Other cues common in neurocritical care are decreased ventilatory and/or circulatory adaptive capacity, decreased responsiveness (confused to absent verbal response plus absence of ability to follow commands), pain, and mobility-restricting therapeutic devices (such as orthopedic splints and pins and invasive cannulae in limbs).

HYPOTHESIS TESTING

The large diagnostic categories described previously are frequently activated even before the first contact with the patient. Observation, examination, and laboratory data all serve to confirm or refute these nursing diagnoses felt to be highly probable on the basis of medical diagnosis and known pathophysiologic states.

Similar reasoning process and use of knowledge packets occur when one is confronted with a change in patient state or a new symptom. Let us take, for example, increased anxiety in a patient with Guillian-Barre syndrome. (Guillian-Barre is a syndrome of ascending polyneuropathy, which can cause symmetrical loss of peripheral nerve innervation to muscles in all limbs, neck and face, thus creating paralysis of voluntary movement of limbs, eyes and face, and of breathing and swallowing. In severe cases loss of function may ascend over hours or days from lower limbs to cranial nerves).

Pre-encounter information is that the patient has had slowly ascending loss of movement of legs and some weakness in the hands and arms. He is in intensive care for close observation and respiratory support is necessary. On change of shift rounds he is restless, says he feels "jumpy" and is afraid to fall asleep. These statements plus his appearance are consistent with the symptom, anxiety.

Differential Diagnosis.   Two primary hypotheses form the start of data search. These are 1) moderate anxiety secondary to uncertainty about progression of disease symptoms and ultimate recovery and 2) moderate anxiety secondary to impending ventilatory insufficiency. Hypothesis 1 comes from the knowledge package about anxiety (vague apprehension of the unknown) coupled with that of the disease process related to the change in body image and progression of loss of motor function. Hypothesis 2 stems from the knowledge of hypoxia (with anxiety and fear of falling asleep as subjective symptoms) and the disease course and neuroanatomy (proximity of thoracic and upper-extremity peripheral nerves at root level with high potential for respiratory and subsequent swallowing involvement). Pre-encounter data tells us that paralysis is ascending and involving upper extremities and that respiratory–ventilatory insufficiency is a risk for this patient. Since hypothesis 2 carries a threat to life, data collection begins with ruling ventilatory sufficiency in or out. Bedside spirometry (with vital capacity at lower levels than before and approaching 25% of normal), observation of the patient's speaking patterns (short sentences with frequent breaths interspersed), and breathing patterns (increased rate, increased use of sternocleidomastoid muscles) provide confirmation of impending ventilatory insufficiency as the primary cause of the symptom, anxiety. Blood gases drawn at this time, but with results not available for some minutes, will confirm the extent of respiratory (oxygen-exchange) insufficiency.

At this point the diagnosis of ventilatory insufficiency is in the shared nursing and medical area of physiologic instability with threat to life. The data confirming the diagnosis is shared with the physician who may then choose further supportive data and who bears authority and responsibility for management of ventilation.

While the ventilatory insufficiency is being managed by medical therapy, the same data provides the basis for the nursing diagnoses: *decreased adaptive capacity, ventilatory, and diminished capacity for self-care secondary to decreased ventilatory reserve,* which leads to *increased fear and anxiety.*

Nursing Management.   Nursing management stemming from this diagnosis involves avoiding or decreasing activities that require increased ventilatory effort—for example self-care activities that involve use of the still mobile upper extremities, turning himself, and emotional arousal. The alternate diagnostic hypothesis (*anxiety secondary to unknown disease progression*) becomes relevant here, as an interaction with the primary cause of anxiety (*i.e., inadequate ventilation*). One presumes most people would be anxious about the rapidity of worsening disease, breathlessness, and the obvious increase in monitoring and concern by the intensive-care staff. One knows this type of anxiety is based in reality and is likely to dissipate as the situation resolves. Therefore, long-term insight therapy is not appropriate, in fact it may increase psychophysiologic arousal. Realistic reassurance that the staff will care for him, will help him breathe and will not let him stop breathing are appropriate management strategies for this situationally based anxiety that interacts with physiologically based anxiety. Decreased self-care capacity is managed by performing daily activities such as toothbrushing, feeding, turning, and dressing.

Prognosis.   Prognosis for resolution of primary symptom (anxiety) with resolution of physiologic instability is based on knowledge of natural course of the disorder and resolution of ventilatory insufficiency with ventilatory assistance. Prognosis of secondary anxiety is variable depending upon the degree to which the patient feels safe in the hands of the staff and the skill and confidence that the nurse feels and conveys to the patient. Prognosis for reduction of physical adaptive demands is excellent if staff perform daily functions for the patient (positioning, bathing, feeding) and anticipate and respond to her changes in comfort.

SUMMARY

Diagnostic reasoning in the neurocritical-care area appears on the surface to be quite different from that in settings where the nurse works with chronically ill persons. However, this chapter illustrates the commonality of thinking processes with those described in previous chapters. Knowledge of pathophysiology of the disease process interacts with knowledge of the problems common to patients in the setting (or with a given state of health or illness), the responses of the individual, and the characteristics of the individual. Clustering of cues activate the hypothesis of a *general* category of diagnosis and further data search narrows the possibilities to two or three *highly probable* diagnoses. Degree of *risk* to the patient's *psychophysiologic integrity* determines the priority of establishing the differential diagnosis.

BIBLIOGRAPHY

Aspinall MJ: Nursing diagnosis: the weak link. Nursing Outlook 24:433–437, 1976

Benoliel J, McCorkle R and Young K: Development of a social dependency scale. Research in Nursing and Health 3:3–10, 1980

Gordon M: Predictive strategies in diagnostic tasks. Nursing Research 29:39–45, 1980

Castles MR: Interrater agreement in the use of nursing diagnosis. In Kim MJ and Moritz DA: Classification of Nursing Diagnosis: pp. 153–158 Proceedings of the Third and Fourth National Conferences. NY: McGraw-Hill, 1982

Grier MR: Decision making about patient care. Nursing Research 25:105–110, Mar-Apr, 1976

Hansen AC and Thomas DB: A conceptualization of decision-making. Nursing Research 17:436–443, Sept-Oct 1968

Mitchell PH: Neurologic Disorders. In Kinney M et al. AACN Clinical Reference for Critical Care Nursing, NY: McGraw-Hill, 1980

Mitchell P et al: Neurological Assessment for Nursing Practice. Reston, Va.: Reston Publishing Co, 1984 (in press)

Orem D: Nursing: Concepts of Care 3rd ed., NY: McGraw-Hill, 1980

CHAPTER NINE

Clinical Examples: A Comparison

Pamela H. Mitchell

The foregoing chapters have emerged from the thinking of four practitioners of nursing, each working with people who have distinctly different medical diagnoses. It is evident, however, that phenomena of concern to nursing cut across these patient groups. Pain, fatigue, support systems, relationships, sleep disturbance, body image, and loss of control are areas of nursing diagnosis that were found among the groups of patients and clients seen by these clinicians. All chapters clearly showed, through examples, that the nurse is seeking data to guide understanding of the impact of pathophysiologic state on the quality of daily living and capacity for self-care (the nursing domain) rather than data that guides diagnosis and direct management of the pathologic state itself (the medical domain).

The *process* by which each clinician came to nursing diagnosis is just as Tanner predicted in her description of the use of data by experts versus novice nurses. Each of the clinicians in this section postulates a *general diagnostic category* as the initial hypothesis, for example: sexual difficulty, respiratory problem, activity tolerance problem. This general hypothesis serves to guide the data search by narrowing it to two or three specific diagnostic possibilities and then by testing these possibilities. Mitchell, Blainey, and McCorkle provide examples of this differential diagnostic process in three settings.

Another common feature of these chapters is the strong influence of *setting* and *specialty* on the formulation of general diagnostic categories and on the selection of areas for an early data search. McCorkle, Simmons, and Mitchell each list five to nine diagnostic categories common to their client or patient population. Even though they do not explicitly state this, the relatively small number of categories (or knowledge "chunks") is exactly what is predicted by short-term memory theory (see Chapter 3). The content of these knowledge packets is shaped by experience with people in that given clinical setting. For the experienced nurse, knowledge of the setting and a specialized client-patient group allows one to immediately narrow the range of possible nursing diagnoses from infinity to a manageable few. When studying diagnostic reasoning in practicing nurses, Gordon (1981) remarked on the frequency with which subjects requested seemingly irrelevant contextual cues. It is likely that these contextual (setting) cues, while irrelevant to a given symptom, are extremely useful to the nurse when consolidating the potential data search field into a manageable size.

Premature closure and, thus, nonconsideration of alternative diagnoses is, of course, the danger of using setting and specialty exclusively in structuring the data field. In Chapter 9, a system is described by which a clinician may review categories of function by priority in order to avoid premature closure.

As intended by the editors, the chapters in this section do illustrate the commonality of diagnostic reasoning in experienced practitioners. They also illustrate the *differences in content of knowledge packets* that are a function of setting interacting with the biomedical state of the person. For example, Blainey, McCorkle and Simmons work with people who have chronic, incurable diseases. However, the nursing diagnoses and categories of priority concern differ among these client groups, as a function of setting (outpatient clinic, home, treatment center) interacting with the trajectory of the disease state and treatment regimen. McCorkle's and Blainey's focus is on diagnoses that guide symptom management. However, McCorkle's clients are in their own homes, and often facing death. Thus, she gears her thinking to determining the nature of obstacles that thwart the abilities of persons to bring satisfactory closure to daily living, while Blainey seeks to determine obstacles that thwart the quality of ongoing daily living. Although Simmons is involved with people who are potentially terminally ill, a treatment (renal dialysis) both provides promise for continued life and places extra demands on daily living for the patient. The areas of diagnostic concern that she describes incorporate both the treatment and disease-related demands on daily living. The impact of technology on demands of daily living is also evident in Mitchell's description of nursing diagnostic areas in critical care. The sophisticated monitoring equipment provides additional data for the nurse to use, and at the same time creates additional demands in terms of noise, personnel, and restrictions on body position.

A final difference among chapters is in the precision of specificity of nursing diagnostic statements. Although the categories, or areas of nursing diagnosis, are consistent with those identified by the

National Conference groups (Kim and Moritz, 1982), none are stated in precisely the same terms as the "approved" diagnoses. This discrepancy should not be taken as a criticism of the authors, for the conference group listings are by no means complete, nor do they provide specific diagnostic statements within the broad categories so far defined. As Woods notes in the next section of this book, development of a taxonomy (classification) of nursing diagnoses proceeds by both inductive and deductive reasoning. The diagnostic processes described by these authors have proceeded inductively, deriving from the accumulated experience and thoughtful reflection of practitioners. Mitchell attempts to bring the diagnostic possibilities in critical care down to a manageable few by using larger conceptual categories such as physiologic stability and adaptive capacity. Such categorization provides some measure of deductive reasoning. It is our belief that the classification of nursing diagnoses will proceed most readily from this kind of movement back and forth between empirically derived clinician diagnoses, tested against theoretical formulations.

EXAMINING ONE'S OWN DIAGNOSTIC REASONING

These chapters have served as examples of the way in which four clinicians approach the diagnostic reasoning process. How can individual nurses examine their own reasoning processes in order to refine their approach to nursing diagnosis? Read these chapters and compare the settings and clientele to your own. If they are similar, ask if these ideas "fit" with your experience. What other common problems or diagnostic categories have you found in your experience?

If the examples are quite different from your own setting, use the examples for the process of reasoning, and compare the content of your knowledge base using the following set of questions:

- ☐ What are the common problems in daily living in the patients or clients with whom I work?
- ☐ How does the setting influence what I notice? Are there certain pieces of information I make certain to know about before I even visit the patient (client)?
- ☐ How do I make my first contacts? What are the questions or observations I make first?
- ☐ When a patient or client presents a new problem or symptom, what are the first possible causes that come

to mind? How many are there that I usually consider? How does this shape the kind of information I seek next?

☐ How do I avoid premature closure? Do I have a system to avoid jumping to conclusions?

☐ Do my interventions follow logically from the diagnoses I make? If I find myself intervening without diagnosis, can I "back up" and make the "intuitive" diagnosis explicit?

Examining one's own diagnostic reasoning processes is extremely hard work. The authors of these chapters worked for a very long time to make their reasoning explicit to themselves and to each other. They did not work in isolation, but talked and argued with each other. They believe the end product enables them to better teach others how to make nursing diagnoses, and to make better diagnoses themselves. A similar process should be helpful to practicing nurses as they seek to improve their own diagnostic skills.

BIBLIOGRAPHY

Gordon, M.: Predictive strategies in the diagnostic tasks. *Nursing Research* 29:39–45, Jan –Feb 1980

Kim, M.J. and Moritz, D.A.: *Classification of Nursing Diagnoses: Proceedings of the Third and Fourth National Conferences.* NY: McGraw-Hill, 1982

SECTION FOUR

Taxonomies and Technology: Future Directions for Diagnostic Reasoning in Nursing

Nancy F. Woods

Introduction

Over the last two decades, nurses have made considerable progress in defining the processes they employ in decision-making. Nursing curricula and nursing texts reflect concern with an increasingly sophisticated data base. Nursing's approach to assessment has included integration of physical assessment and biomedical data with information related to daily living and developmental tasks. It involves environment for daily living in health-related areas and external resources available to, or needed by, the person or family as well as refined approaches to gathering information about intrapersonal and social phenomena influencing health. In addition, several individuals and groups have made major contributions to the descriptions of phenomena of concern in the nursing field by developing classification systems of nursing diagnoses. Processes by which diagnoses are made are becoming more apparent in both nursing texts and in courses of study.

This section will focus on three areas of development for the future. The first chapter deals with the development of a taxonomy for nursing, an essential step in refining decision-making in nursing. The notions of taxonomy and classification system will be discussed. Both inductive and deductive approaches to the development of a taxonomy will be considered. The second chapter includes consideration of models for studying diagnostic reasoning in nursing. Approaches employing computer-assisted decision making will be considered. The third chapter addresses the development of computer simulations for teaching diagnostic reasoning and emphasizes the integration of the unique requirements of nursing versus other disciplines.

CHAPTER TEN

Toward a Taxonomy of Nursing Phenomena

Nancy F. Woods

The nature and range of diagnostic categories within nursing, or any other practice discipline, influence all elements of the diagnostic and decision making processes. The phenomena of concern to nursing and the theories that describe and explain them

> shape the data search field by influencing which cues nurses will notice and the significance that will be attached to them; determine which descriptive or explanatory hypotheses will be activated by the presenting data; provide an organizing image essential for the storage and retrieval of information for diagnosis and decision making; determine prognostic areas and variables that serve as predictors of prognosis; influence the rationale for prescription of nursing actions; and determine the nature of responses that may be anticipated when nursing actions have been undertaken.

It can be readily appreciated that naming and describing the phenomena of concern to nursing are essential, not only to the decision-making processes employed by clinicians, but also to the advancement of theory building that shapes future clinical judgments and decisions.

Although several individuals and groups are in the process of developing classification systems of nursing diagnoses or problems there is not yet widespread acceptance of a single approach, or an overall conceptual framework. Within the next decade or two, it will be essential for nurses to devise a taxonomy of those phenomena that are of primary concern to nursing's practice and scholarship.

TAXONOMY

The terms taxonomy and classification system are frequently used interchangeably but within this context it is important to distinguish between them. *Taxonomy* is the science of classification; it deals with division of phenomena into systematic groupings that form categories, and is usually related to the principles or laws of a discipline. Each group characterized by common attributes and constituting a category is called a *taxon*. The process of classification, by contrast, involves the assignment of things to a category.

The processes of identifying, describing and grouping phenomena into a unified category system is characteristic of the early phases of the development of a science, and is discussed by some as the development of taxonomic or naming theory. (Dickoff and James, 1968; Northrup 1959). Classification, by definition, is concerned with arranging or distributing phenomena into classes. It is clearly only one of the processes involved in developing a taxonomy.

DESIRABLE CHARACTERISTICS OF A CLASSIFICATION SYSTEM

There are several characteristics that are desirable, if not essential, in any system of classification:

- ☐ The classification system should be natural or relevant.
- ☐ The set of categories should be exhaustive.
- ☐ The individual categories should be mutually exclusive or disjoint.
- ☐ The category system is derived from and develops a principle of ordering.
- ☐ The individual categories are formulated on the same level of abstraction or discourse.
- ☐ The classification system should be useful.
- ☐ The classification system should be constructable. (Kerlinger, 1973 and Murphy, 1978)

Natural or Relevant

A classification system can be said to be *natural* if it corresponds to the nature or character of the thing being classified. It is *relevant* if it pertains to the phenomena being classified. One of the difficulties encountered when nurses employ medical classification systems, such as the ICDA Manual, for classifying phenomena of concern to nursing practice is that the medical classification system is inadequate for nursing. Although the ICDA is a sophisticated system, the factors it is concerned with are predominately disease entities. The phenomena of concern to nursing includes medical problems and their management, but they constitute only one element in nursing's domain. The nursing domain also incorporates the requirements and resources for managing daily living, developmental tasks, and the environment.

Exhaustive

The set of categories in a classification system is exhaustive when each member of the group to which it applies will fit into one class of the system. This implies that each possible member could be classified, and there would be no residual members who did not fit into the classification scheme. Ideally, nursing phenomena would be viewed in a way that would encompass all the possible diagnoses or problems of concern to nurses. For example, a classification scheme that was concerned with only pathological entities such as deviations in cardiovascular, renal, and gastrointestinal function (to the exclusion of associated problems in managing the activities and demands of daily living) would be inadequate, and certainly would not exhaust the kinds of problems of concern to nursing. To meet the criteria of exhaustiveness, one first considers the broad boundaries of the phenomena to be classified, and then proceeds to group the phenomena. The potential scope is defined by the character of the problems that one seeks to classify. In nursing, the broad boundaries encompass health, daily living, and the elements of the environment in which that daily living occurs.

Disjoint

It is essential that the taxons or classes in any classification system be *disjoint*, or mutually exclusive; that is, no particular case could fail into more than one class. This implies that the classes be sufficiently differentiated. For example, if one were classifying body weight, it would be important to specify rules for inclusion or exclusion regarding the classes.

Classification scheme #1, in Table 10–1, would end in confusion about how to classify anyone whose weight was 100 lbs, 150 lbs or 200 lbs, because the classes overlap. Scheme #2, however, would provide a mutually exclusive system as long as the weights were given in whole numbers. One can appreciate the need for finer class bound-

Table 10-1

A Comparison of Two Classification Systems for Weight Measurements

Classification Scheme #1	Classification Scheme #2
0–100 lbs	0–99 lbs
100–150 lbs	100–149 lbs
150–200 lbs	150–199 lbs
200–250 lbs	200–249 lbs

aries, or for a decision rule about how to round off weights in the event that they were reported to the second or third decimal place. The confusion in categorization that is possible with even this simple example illustrates the complexity one encounters in classifying more complex phenomena such as nursing diagnoses or problems.

Consider the distinctions between the following categories:

Solitude—being alone without discomfort

Lonesomeness—being alone or with others, but with mild-to-moderate discomfort associated with absence or loss of a desired person or relationship

Loneliness—being alone or with others, but with moderate to severe discomfort associated with absence or loss of a desired person or relationship (Carnevali 1983).

Although the categories are defined clearly, it may be possible to misclassify those individuals who feel moderate discomfort associated with absence or loss.

Ordering to Develop an Underlying Principle

The classification system should be derived from a principle of ordering and should develop that principle. Identification of the appropriate principles for a taxonomy of nursing has been, and will continue to be, a critical phase in the development of a taxonomy that can be embraced by the discipline. Currently, there seem to be many competing principles underlying current classification attempts. The principle of ordering might differ in a taxonomy of nursing diagnosis generated by theorists or researchers versus clinicians. For example, one might classify problems according to body systems as is done in the ICD or one might derive a taxonomy from concepts such as self, role, and environment.

Parallel Levels of Abstraction

The individual categories in a taxonomy should be formulated on the same level of abstraction or discourse. This implies that there exists a parallelism between the taxons and between subclasses. An example of a parallel and non parallel portion of a taxonomy is given in Table 10-2. In the first example, the categories sensory deprivation and sensory overload are parallel, that is, at the same level of abstraction. Both are conditions in which sensory experiences are altered. Their subclasses are parallel, each representing an abstraction about mechanisms by which sensory experiences are altered. In the second example, both deafness and blindness represent altered sensory reception, transmission, and integration, and are therefore not at the same level of abstraction as is altered environmental stimuli. Deafness and blindness both represent subclasses of altered sensory reception.

Usefulness

The classification system should be useful to the discipline and others who might employ it. This implies that the users can under-

Table 10-2
Parallel and Non-Parallel
Structure in Taxonomies

Parallel Structure	Non-Parallel Structure

1.0 Sensory Deprivation
   1.1 Altered environmental stimuli
   1.2 Altered sensory reception, transmission or integration
   1.3 Altered chemical milieu
2.0 Sensory Overload
   2.1 Altered environmental stimuli
   2.2 Altered sensory reception, transmission or integration
   2.3 Altered chemical milieu
	1.0 Sensory Deprivation
	   1.1 Deafness
	
	   1.2 Altered environment
	   1.3 Blindness
	2.0 Sensory Overload

stand the system and find it helpful rather than confusing. Unless the terminology employed in the taxonomy is recognized by the majority of users, the taxonomy may be misused or ignored. Orientation to such a system is essential, particularly where the organization of the taxonomy reflects new concepts or principles.

Constructability

Finally, it is important that the classification system be constructable. The quality of constructability implies that by its very structure, the classification system can be seen to satisfy conditions of exhaustiveness and disjointedness. In other words, the adequacy of the system can be established without examining every possible case. (Murphy 1978).

APPROACHES TO THE DEVELOPMENT OF TAXONOMIES IN NURSING: PRESENT AND FUTURE

Currently there are two important approaches being employed in the development of a taxonomy of nursing diagnoses. These have been labelled inductive and deductive approaches.

Inductive

The inductive approach has included the development of nursing diagnoses from the particular nursing practice experiences of individuals, and the diagnoses generated by this approach have often been classified alphabetically. This approach is similar to that employed by biologists, who observed many entities in nature, and then began to classify them. Groups who have employed the inductive approach to enumerating nursing diagnoses usually begin by generating a large list of problems that particular populations of individuals experience. Once these diagnoses are labelled and defined, they can be validated in clinical practice. Suppose the population in question consists of patients who are experiencing neurological problems. Nurses would begin by making an exhaustive list of diagnoses the patients experienced. These diagnoses would then be subjected to clinical validation to ascertain whether they were important in this area of practice. It would not be unusual for these diagnoses to be clustered in the areas of physical, cognitive, affective, and social function. Categorizing these diagnoses, however, would be difficult because many of them could be subsumed under more than one class.

For example, a diagnosis of confusion might well be attributable to physiological causes, such as electrolyte imbalance, or to alterations in the person's usual environment brought about by admission to an intensive-care unit. A final step in the inductive approach can be the development of a conceptual framework consistent with the identified diagnosis.

The following example is an illustration of a diagnostic-concept, alteration of control in daily living, generated by the inductive method. An overview of the concept is presented, followed by a discussion of risk factors, populations at risk, manifestations, areas of loss-of-control in daily living, a dynamic description of the concept, and complications of the diagnosis.

LOSS OF CONTROL IN DAILY LIVING*

Overview: A presenting situation in which the individual or family no longer have, or feel they have, the freedom or ability to make decisions or manage themselves and their own functions, their lifestyle, their relationships with others, their space

Risk Factors: ☐ Being young or old

☐ Being distant from one's normal locale (Increased Distance = Decreased Control)

☐ Being deviant from norms of the health-care providers or system (economically, socially, educationally, ethnically, or in one's values)

☐ The number or amount of bodily functions one cannot do for one's self

☐ Being unable to make one's self understood (aphasia, lack of English, confusion, laryngectomy)

(continued on following pages)

* Concept developed by D. Carnevali in collaboration with University of Washington Hospital Clinical Specialists: Barbara Fellows, Enterostomy Therapy; Dale Land, Psychiatry; Janet Loehr, Rehabilitation; Barbara Sherer, Cardiovascular; Joie Whitney, Medical-Surgical.

□ Being infectious, isolated secondary to receiving transplants or radiation

□ Being forced to undergo treatment or demands against one's expressed wishes or without one's consent

□ Accumulation of areas of loss, duration of loss or growing losses in selected areas of control

□ Increased numbers of differing persons providing care

□ Decreased plans for continuity

□ Lack of a provider they identify with

Populations at Risk: Patients, family, staff

Manifestations: *Withdrawal*—speaking and participating less, decreased spontaneity, passivity, lack of participation, weeping

Aggression—use of abusive language toward people seen as having the control, physical violence, verbal violence, refusal to participate in prescribed activities

Development of nonproductive or counterproductive strategies to try to gain some control:

turning on the call light frequently

trying to pit one of the controlling members against another, courting the controlling people or selected members of the group, obsequiousness "nothing is right", constant complaining or focusing complaints on one thing

asks others to serve as self in daily living activities

behavior to make providers adapt to patient's usual pace

makes obvious efforts to keep environment arranged on own terms

Areas for Loss
of Control in
Daily Living

Choice—in eating, times of activity, places one can go, people one can relate to, nature of relationships

Privacy—bodily, space, information on functioning, relationships

Goals—sense of accomplishment
sense of being needed/valuable
sense of competence

Sleep

Sexual functioning: impotence, opportunities for sexual activity

Perspective on life and relationships with others 2° to changes from usual cues sent by others

Usual/preferred patterns of daily living (in or out of hospital)

Usual/preferred relationships with others

Clothing styles

Dynamics:

The individual/family anticipates or actually perceives they are experiencing loss of freedom or ability to manage themselves, their decision making, their lifestyle, their space and their relationships with others. It may result from loss of ability to function (internal loss of control). It may be imposed by others (external loss of control.) It may be a combination of internal and external. The loss can generate internal responses of fear, anxiety, frustration or aggression, with accompanying physiologic manifestations. The external responses will be associated with the skills of the person in compensatory efforts as long as he keeps trying to regain or retain some areas of control or with anger; apathy if he sees little hope of achieving or regaining control.

Complications:

☐ Alienation of support (staff) persons family and loss of external resources

secondary to behavior, deviant from
the norms of the support persons
☐ Depression—suicide—neglect   of
health
☐ Alteration in family relationships secondary to change in control

It can be seen that a whole cluster of highly specific diagnoses
could be generated from this one diagnostic concept, together with
prognostic considerations and treatment protocols. Use of information regarding risk factors and knowledge of presenting situations the
patient or family may have to face could result in the development of
anticipatory diagnoses and sound preventive strategies. Loss of control is a diagnostic concept illustrating a nursing (daily living–health
status) perspective that could intersect with a large number of pathophysiologic–psychopathologic phenomena, treatment regimens, and
treatment environment (situations where the environment itself generates loss of control).

The development of diagnostic concepts for phenomena in the
nursing domain that, in turn, generate logical clusterings of associated diagnoses and treatment protocols is one strategy for developing
a diagnostic taxonomy.

Deductive

The second approach, the deductive approach, involves the
generation of nursing diagnoses from a conceptual model for nursing. Using the conceptual framework for nursing described by
Carnevali (1983), a taxonomy of nursing diagnoses could be developed that is based on the major constructs of health and daily living,
resources and requirements for daily living. Both the inductive and
deductive approaches to generating a taxonomy for nursing are currently proceeding simultaneously, and the Fifth National Conference
on Nursing Diagnosis in 1982 reviewed both methods. Arguing for a
deductive approach, Roy (1981) points out that the alphabetical system may be an adequate organizing principle for an index or phone
book, but it does not demonstrate a given order to parts, it does not
show the relationship between parts, nor does it allow us to discern
the absence of parts. She further recommends that the organizing
principle for our diagnostic classification system reflect our image of
nursing's domain of practice, including our view of the nature of the
person, the goal of nursing action, and interventions nurses use.

Using Rogers' concept of unitary man, participants in the Fifth National Conference explored the relationship between the nursing diagnosis generated by previous conference groups and the patterns of unitary man. Unitary man, as distinct from "biological" man and "social" man, refers to a human being that cannot be known by knowing the parts. Unitary man is an open system, an energy field. According to Rogers, developmental process pertains to the negentropic nature of human systems (growing in diversity). Development is always emerging. Man and the environment are constantly evolving in mutual simultaneous interaction. Change is continuous. Development becomes more complex in pattern and organization. Change occurs rhythmically, and the rhythmicities in open systems are spiraling and nonrepeating. The similarity in rhythmicities make prediction possible, and thus the likelihood that rhythmic patterns may be altered. Patterns of unitary man that can provide a specific framework for the generation of nursing diagnosis include: wakefulness, activity, communication, relationships, knowing, material exchange, valuing, and choosing, or deliberate goal-setting. Within each of these patterns, the duration, rate, or amount may vary. Hypo- and hypervigilance, and altered levels of consciousness are diagnostic labels related to wakefulness.

Kim (1981) predicts convergence of these two approaches (but not complete convergence) around the year 2000. In the intervening years, the challenge to develop a classification system remains pivotal to progress in diagnostic reasoning in the nursing domain. Without a taxonomy that adequately reflects the concerns of the discipline, it will be difficult, if not impossible, to participate in more sophisticated forms of decision-making and to transmit these processes to students and clinicians in nursing and other disciplines.

BIBLIOGRAPHY

American Nurses' Association. *A Social Policy Statement*. Kansas City, Kansas, American Nurses Association, 1980

Bircher, A: The Concept of Nursing Diagnosis. In Classification of Nursing Diagnosis. Proceedings of the 3rd and 4th National Conferences. Kim M and Moritz D (eds), New York: McGraw-Hill Book Co, 1982

Carnevali D: Nursing Care Planning: Diagnosis and Management, 3rd ed. Philadelphia, JB Lippincott Co, 1983

Dickoff J and James P: A Theory of Theories: A Position Paper. Nursing Research 17:197–203, 1968

Hangartner C: Principles of Classification in First National Conference for Classification of Nursing Diagnosis. St. Louis, CV Mosby and Co, 1973

Kerlinger F: Foundations of Behavioral Research. New York, Holt, Rinehart & Winston Inc, 1973

Kim M: Issues Related to Research on the Classification of Nursing Diagnosis pp 124–137. In Kim and Moritz, *op cit.*

Murphy E: The Logic of Medicine. Baltimore: The Johns Hopkins University Press, 1978

Northrop FC: The Logic of the Sciences and the Humanities. 1959

Roy Sr. Callista: Historical Perspective of the Theoretical Framework for the Classification of Nursing Diagnosis pp. 235–249. In Kim and Moritz, *op cit.*

CHAPTER 11

Methods for Studying Diagnostic Reasoning in Nursing

Nancy F. Woods

Diagnostic reasoning in nursing practice can be investigated from the perspectives reflected in theory and research on problem-solving, judgement, and decision-making. Although each of these perspectives contributes to an improved understanding of diagnostic reasoning, each has a different emphasis. Studies of problem-solving emphasize the process by which an individual or a group produces a solution. Studies of judgment typically emphasize the evaluation or categorizing of phenomena. Studies of decision-making are concerned with describing or prescribing how individuals choose a course of action when there are several alternatives available as well as a variable amount of knowledge about the possible outcomes of these alternatives. Clinical reasoning involves judgment, as in the use of cognitive processes to make a diagnosis, and problem-solving or decision about consequent outcomes or courses of action. Clinical decision-making must be concerned with prescriptive decision analyses; that is, the ways people *should* make a choice, as well as descriptive decision analyses, *how* people do make a choice.

This chapter will examine general approaches to studying diagnostic reasoning in nursing practice. Ultimate outcomes of these studies include a better understanding of reasoning processes, improved skill of individual clinicians, and ability to predict and control outcomes associated with diagnostic reasoning.

Elstein has identified two general approaches to studying judgment and thinking that emanate from the literatures of organizational psychology, cognitive psychology, and statistics. The first approach emphasizes the intellectual processes employed by individuals as they make judgments or decisions or solve problems. The second approach emphasizes the modeling of the judgment or decision through studying input–output relations. The aims of these two major approaches, their positions regarding the use of introspective data, their emphasis on understanding or prediction as the primary aim of inquiry, and the role of mathematical modeling are summarized in Table 11–1. Each of these approaches and its potential contribution to the study of diagnostic reasoning in nursing will be discussed in more detail.

STUDIES OF INFORMATION PROCESSING

Studies whose aim is to further understand the processes by which nurses reach judgments and solve problems can add to a general explanation of human thought processes. These studies frequently focus on information processing by individuals and thus may be referred to as "process-tracing" studies. They may focus on a large and complex task, on a simple task, or on part of a task. Their aim is to observe the process of thinking in an environment that closely resembles the real task setting. Some studies of this genre rely on verbal reports of the rules or algorithms used to generate the judgment or decision. The approaches used include: having the individual dictate aloud the processes employed in categorizing cases into various diagnostic categories, or using an approach analogous to the

Table 11–1

	Information Processing	Modelling Input/Output Relations
Aim of approach	understanding of process by which humans reach judgments	describe, explain decision-making
Introspective data	legitimate data source	not legitimate data source
Relative importance of understanding and prediction	understanding greater than prediction	prediction greater than understanding
Role of mathematical modeling	confirmatory analyses	central to analyses

game "Twenty Questions," in which the individual is allowed to ask a sequence of questions for further information. This approach has been challenged by some who argue that the actual process of thinking out loud alters the process and content of thinking. Process-tracing studies can be used to trace the approaches to diagnostic reasoning employed by experts and novice nurses. Examples such as those included in Chapters 3 and 4 illustrate the differences in processes that might be revealed by contrasting two groups of nurses.

Other approaches of this genre include in-basket, programmed patient, and tab-item methods. In *in-basket* approach entails providing an individual with several sources of information, such as documents in an incoming mail basket, to which an individual must make responses (decisions). *Programmed patients* are actresses or actors who have been trained to present a clinical case history for diagnosis. The *tab-item method* involves giving a clinical problem along with a list of several tests or sources of information. Next to each item is a tab covering the information gained by that test or line of questioning. By removing the tabs, the individual leaves a record of the approaches she or he has taken. This process could be employed easily using a computer to offer choices and record the reasoning process. (see Chapter 12) More complex variations on this approach can be employed, including the derivation of weighted goals where positive weights are assigned to those items that should be included in a thorough assessment and where negative weights are assigned to those that are unnecessary or contraindicated.

Each of these approaches can be applied to studying diagnostic reasoning processes employed by nurses. There are definite strengths associated with these methods, most notably their abilities to further an understanding of human thought processes as opposed to a mere predicting of outcomes or decisions. *Understanding* thought processes implies that one can explain mechanisms producing the diagnostic decision. *Prediction* implies that, given a set of cues, one can make some probabilistic statement about the most likely diagnosis. Prediction of the occurence of phenomena can exist in the absence of understanding of the process or mechanism producing that process. In order to generate a model of information processing, methods such as process-tracing are essential. The limitations of the information processing include methods emphasizing their reliance on subjective, introspective data that cannot, by their very nature, be available to the investigator from any other source. The fact that the subjects report the processes they employ in diagnostic reasoning may actually alter the processes they use. That is, making verbal reports of the processes may require somewhat different cognitive processes than are typically employed in arriving at a diagnosis without verbal reporting. Finally, the results of the genre of studies are not immediately applicable when developing means to improve diagnostic reasoning in complex situations. Table 11–2 summarizes the strengths and limitations of the information-processing perspective.

MODELING
INPUT–OUTPUT RELATIONS

Methods that emphasize input–output relations in modeling decision-making constitute a description of decision-making and its ability to predict and control outcomes.

The decisions nurses and other clinicians make can be classified according to the knowledge they have about factors influencing potential outcomes for any given action. There can be *decisions of certainty*, where each alternative has a specified outcome, *decisions of risk or uncertainty*, where each alternative has a set of possible outcomes, each with some probability of occurence, and *decisions of ignorance*, in which each alternative action has a range of possible outcomes, but the likelihood of each outcome is unknown. Few nursing diagnostic decisions are made under conditions of absolute certainty. More commonly, decisions are made when related outcomes are probabilistic or when the choice must be made between alternatives whose outcomes are unknown. There are two general approaches to modeling judgment that rely on a statistical rule for combining inputs into a decision with more accuracy and consistency than human decision-makers can

Table 11–2
Strengths and Limitations of Methods
Emphasizing Information Processing

Strengths	*Limitations*
furthers understanding and explanation of human thought processes	reliance on subjective, introspective data
essential for the development of an information processing model	reporting of the process may actually alter the processes used in diagnostic reasoning
	results not readily applicable to developing means for assisting decision-making in complex situations

yield. One approach involves using a regression model to estimate weights or probabilities for a group of variables or predictors that simulates the way in which a given individual processes information. The second approach relies on the Bayesian Theorem and is used to describe changes in an individual's judgment when given new information.

MODELING CUES USED IN CLINICAL JUDGMENT

Regression models allow an investigator to present a group of variables or cues to an individual or several individuals who are then asked to select and weigh them, arriving at a clinical judgment. The investigator can subsequently derive a mathematical model that reflects the cues used by the clinicians and their relative importance. These models typically take the form of:

$$Y = a + b_1X_1 + b_2X_2 + \cdots + b_nX_n$$

where Y is the diagnostic outcome;

X_1 is the first cue,

X_2 is the second cue,

X_n is the nth cue,

and

b_1 through b_n are the weights assigned to cues X_1 through X_n

Results of a hypothetical analysis of the relative importance of cues used in diagnosing abdominal pain might be depicted as in Figure 11–1. Suppose the universe of possible cues included verbal complaint of pain, guarding of abdomen, sweating, pallor, rapid pulse, absence of bowel sounds, and abdominal distention. In this example, all cues except the verbal complaint and abdominal guarding are trivial and contribute little to the diagnosis.

Although the regression model approach is useful in arriving at patterns in the use of cues, it has some limitations. First, because of the statistical assumptions necessary for computation of the weights of the cues, it is only possible to use this procedure when the cues are uncorrelated. In our example, pallor, sweating, and rapid pulse are likely to be correlated, thus making estimates of the weights inaccurate.

Regression models cannot be interpreted as true models of the individual's own information-processing strategies. It is possible that an individual may not have used a given item at all in arriving at a

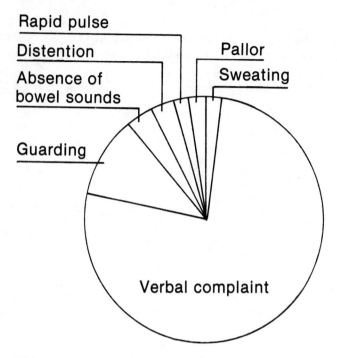

FIG.11–1.   *Relative importance of cues in diagnosing abdominal pain.*

judgment despite the fact that the item is assigned a specific weight in a mathematical model.

The Lens Model.   Another approach to studying decision-making that employs mathematical modeling is referred to as the lens model. The goal of this model is to represent judgment in real situations. The lens model, as applied to the nurse-patient situation, includes

the patient state (PS),

cues related to that state (C),

an inference (I) made about the PS,

actions taken by the nurse (A), and

a goal (G).

The relationships between the components of the model are shown in Figure 11–2 by the lines connecting the components. To date, most of the emphasis in nursing research has been on the left side of the model—the relationships between diagnostic cues and

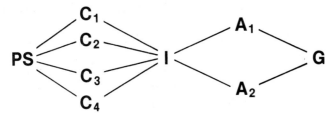

FIG.11–2. *A lens model is applied to the nurse-patient situation. PS = patient state, $C_1 \ldots C_4$ = cues, I = inference, $A_1 \ldots A_2$ = actions, G = goal.*

inferences. Further exploration of this area is essential as is study of the relationships between actions and outcomes.

A more detailed analysis of the left side of Figure 11–2 is given in Figure 11–3. This model expresses relationships between cues, criterion states, and inferences. The left portion of the model depicts the task system, the right, the cognitive system. Each cue is related to the criterion value and to the judgment of the criterion value. Correlations express the relationship between observed cues, the nonobservable criterion states, and the clinician's judgment. For example, r1c to r4c represents correlations between cues 1 through 4 and the criterion, sometimes referred to as the ecological validity of the cues. It is also possible to correlate the r1j through r4j with the clinician's judgment to give the clinician's utilization coefficient for the cues.

Suppose the criterion is energy deficit as judged by several expert clinicians. Cues could include:

C_1: persistent fatigue
C_2: role overload @ work and home
C_3: limited sleep opportunity

In this example, r1c represents how well c1 relates to the criterion (Yc)

Criterion	r1c	C_1	r1j	clinician
Value	r2c	C_2	r2j	judgment
Y_C	r3c	C_3	r3j	Y_j
	r4c	C_4	r4j	

FIG.11–3.

and r1j represents to what extent the clinician uses cue C1 in making her judgment (Yj).

Accuracy of the judgment is limited by the degree of correspondence between the actual criterion values and the real life estimates of these. In addition, the degree of correspondence between the clinician's actual and predicted judgments (cognitive control over the utilization of knowledge) limit the accuracy of judgment.

Finally, the degree to which predicted values for the clinician's judgments correspond with the predicted criterion values represents knowledge of the properties of the task. To improve judgments one can improve the knowledge of the task or the consistency with which existing knowledge is utilized. Lens-model feedback can be used to improve multiple cue probability learning (MCPL). MCPL requires clinicians to make judgments based on values for many cues that are probabilistically related to a criterion. The lens-model-feedback process withholds feedback until sufficient judgments have been made to permit a model of the clinician's judgment policy. The clinician is given a graphic display of her own model of judgment as compared with an ideal.

MODELING CHANGES IN JUDGMENT

The modeling of changes in judgment given new information uses Bayes' theorem, a mathematical formula for calculating the probability of a diagnosis given the presence or absence of a certain piece of information. The application of Bayes' theorem requires information about the probability associated with the diagnosis, which may be derived from a subjective estimate or objective measurement of rates of the diagnosis. The reliability and relevance of the information are also important. Application of Bayes' theorem allows one to calculate how the information should be aggregated to produce a new diagnosis.*

The following discussion illustrates how the Bayesian model can be applied to clinical decision-making. The decision problem includes a series of alternative diagnoses and an outcome value for each alter-

---

* Bayes' theorem (after the Rev. Thomas Bayes) can be used to assist us in attempting to compute the probability of a certain disease or diagnosis (D), given the observed symptom complex (S). Because $P(S) = P(S \text{ and } D) + P(S \text{ and } \bar{D})$, it can be shown mathematically that:

$$(PD/S) = \frac{P(D) \cdot P(S/D)}{P(D) \cdot P(S/D) + P(\bar{D}) \cdot P(S/\bar{D})}$$

native that depends on the likelihood of its occurence and its value to the decision-maker. Each alternative, then, is associated with a set of possible outcomes, and each expected outcome is the product of the likelihood of its occurence and the desirability (or utility) of the outcome. The solution involves finding the alternative for which the outcome is of maximal value.

Problem formulation for decision-making under risk typically involves the construction of a matrix or a decision tree. The decision matrix usually displays the alternatives (A_1 to A_m) on the ordinate and the states of nature, circumstances, or cues, ($S_1 \ldots S_n$, those factors influencing the outcome for a given action) on the abscissa. (See Table 11–3) States of nature might be thought of as states of the client. Alternatives are those diagnoses that generate outcomes—in the case of nursing, possible interventions or prognoses. The outcomes (O_1 to $O_{m,n}$) are then given in the place where the ordinate and abscissa intersect. Outcomes can be thought of as effects of the nursing diagnosis. Each outcome would be assigned a probability and a value by the decision-maker. The probability of each outcome can be specified subjectively by experts in the field, or systematically and objectively by investigations of the phenomenon. The probability of each outcome is given in the matrix as P, such that the probability associated with $O_{1,1}$ is $O_{1,1}/P_1$. The utility (or value) associated with each outcome is given in the matrix as U, such that the probability associated with $O_{1,2}$ is $O_{1,2}/P_2$. (See Table 11–3) The expected utility for each alternative (A_1 to A_m) is the sum of the products of the probability and utility for all the possible outcomes of that action:

Expected utility = $(U_{1,1} P_1) + (U_{1,2} P_2) + \ldots (U_{1,n} P_n)$.

Table 11–3
Formulation of a Decision Under Risk Problem: Matrix

Diagnostic Alternatives	States or Cues (S)		
	S_1	$S_2 \ldots S_n$	
A_1	$O_{1,1}/P_1. U_{1,1}$	$O_{1,2}/P_2. U_{1,2}$	$O_{1,n}/P_n. U_{1,n}$
A_2			
.			
.			
.			
A_m	$O_{m,n}/P_n. U_{m,n}$		

To solve the decision problem, one must find which alternative gives the maximal expected utility.

Suppose that a 25-year-old female client comes to the women's health clinic with complaints of lower abdominal cramping. There is a 50% chance that she will begin her menstrual period within a 2-day period. There is a 50% chance that she may be pregnant. The diagnostic alternatives would lead to very different treatment approaches.

Presenting Situation: 25-year-old Female, Sexually Active, with Intermittent Cramping in Lower Abdomen

Diagnostic Alternative	Status	
	Menstruation starts (S_1)	Menstruation doesn't start (S_2)
Dysmenorrhea (A_1)	Correct dx	Incorrect dx
Threatened Abortion (A_2)	Incorrect dx	Correct dx

Course of Events	Outcome	Value
A_1 and S_1	Correct dx ($O_{1,1}$)	1.0
A_2 and S_1	Incorrect dx ($O_{2,1}$) Unnecessary discomfort if analgesia withheld	0.3
A_1 and S_2	Incorrect dx ($O_{1,2}$) Treatment may be teratogenic to embryo	0.0
A_2 and S_2	Correct dx ($O_{2,2}$)	1.0

Each of the diagnostic judgments combined with subsequent events creates an associated outcome. Suppose we assign the following values to the outcomes based on the assumption that unnecessary discomfort is less objectionable to this woman than teratogenicity or malformation of the embryo. Let 1.0 represent the most desirable outcome and 0.0 the least.

Our matrix now looks like this:

	$S_1 = 0.5$	$S_2 = 0.5$
A_1 (dysmenorrhea)	(1.0)	(0.0)
A_2 (abortion)	(0.3)	(1.0)

Now we can calculate the utility associated with each alternative.

$$A_1 = (1.0 \times 0.5) + (0.0 \times 0.5) = .5 + 0 = .5$$
$$A_2 = (0.3 \times 0.5) + (1.0 \times 0.5) = .15 + .5 = .65$$

We can see from this example that the greater utility (.65) is associated with opting for diagnosis A_2 (threatened abortion). If the probabilities associated with the cues were to change, then so would the expected utility of each alternative.

Tree diagrams can also be used to represent the problems of decision-making under risk. The usual convention is to let the initial branches of the tree represent possible actions, and subsequent branches lead to possible outcomes dependent on states of nature. The tree for a problem with two alternatives and two states of nature would look like this:

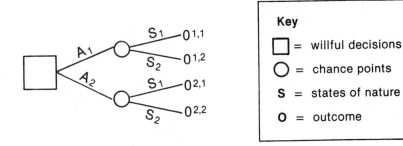

Key	
☐	= willful decisions
○	= chance points
S	= states of nature
O	= outcome

The squares are used to reflect willful decisions, and the circles denote chance points in the problem. One can easily appreciate that the tree would be considerably larger for decisions where multiple alternatives and states of nature exist.

We have seen that decision problems involve consideration of states of nature, diagnostic alternatives, outcomes, probability, and utility functions. In clinical practice, decisions are usually based on an incomplete specification of the alternatives and outcomes. Moreover the accuracy of probability estimates constitute a major source of worry for those making clinical decisions. Probability estimates can be obtained from studies of large samples of the population, or from a survey of experts, but these are statements about the *average*, and their applicability to an individual depends on the extent to which that individual resembles the "average" case. In addition, decisions made within nursing practice are rarely isolated as in the examples we have considered. Multiple decisions that influence one another are made in the course of a single encounter with an individual client (see Table 11–4).

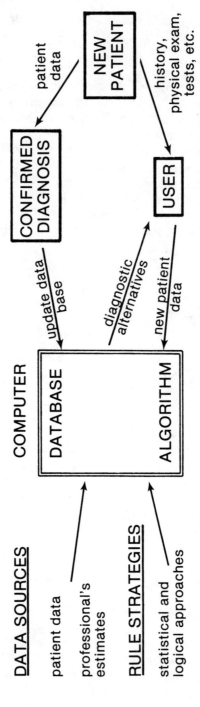

FIG.11–4. Computer–Aided Diagnostic System; A Typical Configuration (after Rogers, Ryack, Moeller 1981)

204

Table 11–4

Strengths and Limits of Methods Emphasizing Input/Output Relations

Strengths	Limitations
Application to teaching decision-making in complex situations	Probabilities may not be available for required parameters
Relies on objective data	Does not illuminate cognitive processes employed in diagnosis
Relationships can be replicated	

COMPUTER ASSISTANCE IN DECISION-MAKING

Because the *gap* between the amount of information available for diagnosis and that accessible from the diagnosticians' memories is so large, computer-based systems are proving useful in the diagnostic process. Computers are capable of storing large quantities of data over time, they can recall stored data, can perform complex logical and mathematical operations at high speed, and can display many diagnostic possibilities, thus assisting humans with their limited capacity for short-term memory.

The basic configuration of a computer-assisted system includes several components:

the computer data base,

the computer algorithm, and

an interactive program for communication between the machine and human

(Rogers, Ryack and Moeller, 1981—see Figure 11–4)

The computer data base for medicine typically consists of disease–symptom relationships, disease probabilities, and other information pertinent to diagnosis and treatment. The algorithm consists of the logical or statistical processes used to derive a solution to the problem from the information included in the data base and information from the history, physical exam, and laboratory tests of the patient currently being treated. These systems cannot be adapted for nursing purposes without considerable modification. Although some medical algorithms overlap with those useful for nursing, there are areas of concern to nurses such as adaptations in daily living developmental tasks and internal and external resources that are not yet adequately represented in those algorithms. In addition, there must be a mechanism for external feedback to allow for assessment of the validity of the computer-generated diagnosis.

The computer algorithm is central to the diagnostic program, and is usually statistical or logical in nature. Statistical algorithms are those which estimate the most likely diagnosis from an analysis of disease-symptom frequencies and disease probabilities. These approaches include the calculation of conditional probabilities based on Bayes' theorem, linear discriminant functions calculated to give the lowest possible probability of misdiagnosis, and matching a patients' profile with all others in the data base or an average symptom profile representative of each disease in the data base.

Logical algorithms are those which usually proceed in a branching fashion. At each step in the process, a decision is made using logical reasoning. Flow charts, sequential questioning and decision-tree approaches are examples of logical algorithms.

Two major methods exist for studying diagnostic reasoning. One examines the thinking process as reported or demonstrated by the diagnostician and illustrated in Tanner's chapters in Section 2. The second method examines input (patient data) and output (clinical judgments and decisions). Both have the potential to contribute ultimately to more effective diagnostic behavior in nurses.

In addition, as generally established nursing diagnoses are emerging, so also is the information needed for utilizing mathematical formulations and computer-assisted diagnoses. As research and clinical practice determine the phenomena that fall within the nursing domain, the client states, the diagnostic alternatives, the potential courses of events, the outcomes, and risks and values of treatments, then nursing too can avail itself more effectively of technologic advances. Mathematical formulations and computer-assisted diagnosing can expedite both clinical practice and the teaching of the diagnostic reasoning process.

BIBLIOGRAPHY

Albert Daniel: Decision Theory in Medicine Milbank Memorial Fund Quarterly 56:3:362–401, 1978

Elstein A., Shulman L, Sprafka S: Medical Problem Solving: An Analysis of Clinical Reasoning. Cambridge, Harvard University Press, 1978

Rogers W, Ryack B and Moeller G: Computer Aided Medical Diagnosis: Literature Review. International Journal of Bio-Medical Computing 10:267–289, 1979

CHAPTER TWELVE

Teaching Diagnostic Reasoning in Nursing with Computer Simulation Exercises

Nancy S. Konikow

In the traditional nursing classroom, it is difficult to teach students how to develop diagnostic reasoning skills. Often this kind of teaching occurs in clinical settings when patient care problems arise. Because it is difficult to predict the occurence of certain patient problems, particularly in acute-care settings, learning how to diagnose and treat these problems must occur through other mechanisms. To help students learn diagnostic reasoning as it is applied to selected nervous system problems that are episodic in nature (thus making opportunities to learn about them limited), computer simulation exercises (CSE)* were developed at the University of Washington, Department of Physiological Nursing, Nervous System Nurse Specialist Training Program† to provide students with the experience of collecting data, analyzing it, and selecting interventions about patient-care problems. Simulation exercises have been used in health-care settings to teach decision making to nursing and medical students (Pearson, 1975; McGuire, 1973). Use of simulation in nursing raises the question of whether clinical phenomena encountered by nurses can be simulated for instruction and research purposes.

* In the literature, the term "computer assisted instruction" (CIA) has been used to describe computer simulations, games, totorials or drills. CSE will be used instead of CIA in this chapter.
† Funded by Advanced Nurse Training Program, Division of Nursing. Grant # 2D22 NU 00018-04R, Department of Health and Human Services.

Three purposes of simulation techniques in education are:

to analyze an ongoing situation,
to advance design and development, and
to train humans (Pearson, 1975)

The analysis of ongoing situations includes the behavior of humans, the output of machines, and the efficiency and effectiveness with which humans are achieving their objectives. Machines, systems, and organizations are identified as part of the advancement of design and development. Training humans involves the performances of new and old skills. With the use of computers in education, the learner is able to retrieve information, analyze it, make decisions, receive feedback, and see the consequences of his decisions with simulation exercises. Desirable characteristics of the problems used in medical and nursing simulation have been discussed by McGuire (1973) and Pearson (1981). First, the information given should not be a predigested summary of a patient, but rather the type of information the nurse would elicit from the patient. Second, the exercise should consist of a series of sequential, interdependent decisions that represent various stages of patient assessment. Third, the nurse receives information about the results of each of her decisions so she can base future actions on these decisions. Fourth, several approaches to the problem should be given with variations in feedback for each approach. Once a decision is made, it cannot be retracted because it is harmful or irrelevant.

Computer simulation exercises using case studies of patients with head injury, spinal cord injury, epilepsy, febrile seizures, and meningitis have been developed in the Nervous System Nurse Specialist Training Program. Several advantages of the use of CSE in the program were identified:

□ A "standard set" of patient problems can be created to satisfy the program's specific instructional goals.
□ During the student's clinical rotation, each student may work with different patient populations, *i.e.*, people with Parkinson's disease, multiple sclerosis, or epilepsy. CSE ensures that students are exposed to similar content areas for those situations they may not encounter during their clinical experience.
□ CSE can run whenever a computer is available; thus they are easily adjusted to fit in with a student's variable and busy schedule.

☐ Instructional time can be increased by creating a learning experience for the student without the necessity for a faculty member being present. Faculty members are then about to devote more time to other individual needs of their students.

Advantages of CSE

☐ creates a "standard set" of pt. care problems

☐ exposes students to similar content

☐ adapts to a student's schedule

☐ increases available instructional time

☐ provides a comfortable exposure to computers

☐ actively involves students

☐ easily adapted to a variety of settings

☐ CSE can provide a comfortable exposure to the use of computers, thus introducing students to this use of technology in education.

☐ CSE involves students actively in the learning process (Chambers and Sprecher, 1980), encouraging them to make decisions in realistic situations that they may encounter in the future.

☐ All of the programs can be adapted for use on a microcomputer, therefore expanding their use. A CSE could even be run in a home.

In the past, there have been some disadvantages of developing CSE. These include the difficult and time-consuming process of creating an effective simulation exercise, difficulties in programming the exercise, and simplistic programs that are trivial or obvious. Other problems include the inability of others to use a program because of programming language, content-related differences in teaching, or treatment philosophies (Gapanoff et al, 1982). To avoid some of these problems, a computer programmer collaborated with nursing faculty on our project.

In the following section, the essential steps in development of CSE are described.

THE BEGINNING

The first step in designing CSE usually involves meeting with a computer programmer who might begin by demonstrating CSE. Participating in these CSE provides a general feeling for their overall design, may be fun to do, and might increase the motivation to begin writing one's own. The programmer can provide a "cookbook" (or author's manual), a series of forms for the purpose of transforming the ideas of "computer naive" faculty members into interesting and secure programs (Gaponoff et al, 1982). The cookbook also makes the process of authoring a program as easy as possible and less time consuming for the faculty member. (See Figure 12–1) An author does not need any knowledge of computer programming (Gaponoff et al, 1982). The programmer usually works with the author of the CSE and translates the author's ideas into a workable computer program, thus relieving the author of valuable time spent on programming.

The categories in the available cookbook may be oriented toward physicians, and may not meet the specific needs of a nursing CSE. Writing a nursing-oriented cookbook may be the first step in the process of writing a CSE. In our experience it was necessary to create a nursing oriented cookbook. The first may take considerable time with subsequent efforts being less time consuming.

RESEARCH THE PROJECT

The most effective way to formulate ideas about the content of the CSE often is reviewing literature about the phenomena. A literature review may suggest models to incorporate in the CSE. For example, an epidural hematoma is a type of head injury requiring the learner (student) to work against time to detect a change in the patient's neurological status. The longer she takes to assess and select appropriate interventions, the more the patient's status deteriorates.

Much research can be done in local hospitals or other clinical agencies. We used a county hospital where most of the head trauma cases go. With permission of the physician it is possible to review medical records of all the patients with a specific diagnosis, in our case, epidural hematomas. Data from these records about the patient's clinical course, neurological status, vital signs, laboratory values, arterial blood gases, ICP monitoring, routine medical care, nursing care, and complications are important for the CSE. The second CSE, on spinal cord injury, was based on two case studies.

1. Recap of data

2. Patient status-physical exam findings
    i.e., neurological
       level of consciousness
       motor
       sensory
       cranial nerves
       cerebellar

3. Laboratory tests

4. Diagnostic tests

5. Nursing assessment and intervention(s)

6. Interpretation of neurological exam findings

7. Implications of neurological deficits

8. Patient/family education

9. Discharge planning and teaching

10. Coping with disability

11. Rehabilitative nursing care

12. Community based — primary care

13. Odds and ends — those that don't
    fit into the above

FIG.12–1.   *A cookbook list for CSE*

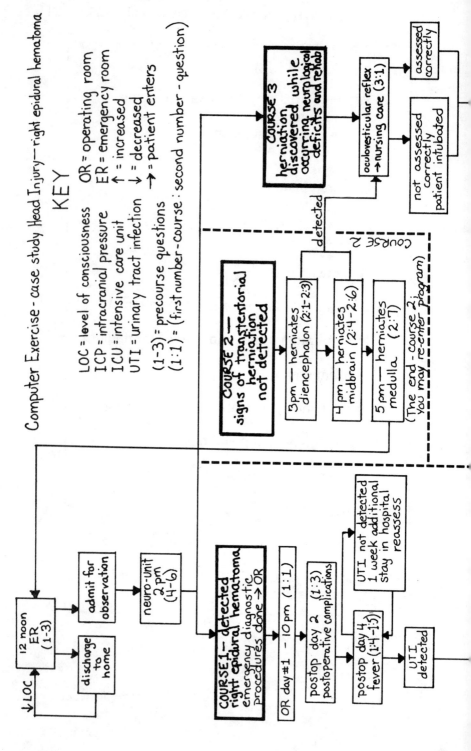

Computer Exercise - case study Head Injury—right epidural hematoma

KEY

LOC = level of consciousness   OR = operating room
ICP = intracranial pressure   ER = emergency room
ICU = intensive care unit   ↑ = increased
UTI = urinary tract infection   ↓ = decreased
                                 → = patient enters

(1-3) = precourse questions
(1:1) = (first number-course : second number - question)

COURSE 3
herniation
discovered while
occurring, neurological
deficits and rehab

oculovesticular reflex
→ nursing care (3:1)

assessed
correctly

not assessed
correctly
patient intubated

detected

COURSE 2
signs of transtentorial
herniation
not detected

3pm — herniates
diencephalon (2:1-2:3)

4pm — herniates
midbrain (2:4-2:6)

5pm — herniates
medulla   (2:7)

(The end - course 2;
you may re-enter program)

COURSE 2

↓ LOC

12 noon
ER
(1-3)

admit for
observation

neuro-unit
2pm
(4-6)

discharge
to
home

COURSE 1— detected
right epidural hematoma
emergency diagnostic
procedures done → OR

OR day#1 - 10pm (1:1)

postop day 2 (1:3)
postoperative complications

postop day 4
fever (1:4-1:5)

UTI not detected
1 week additional
stay in hospital
reassess

UTI
detected

212

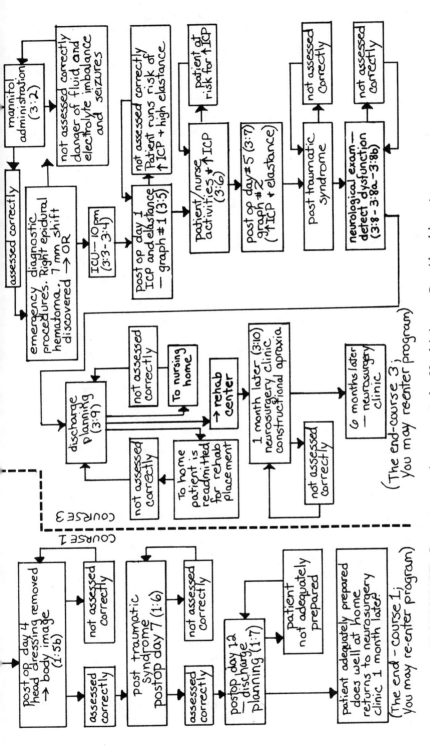

FIG. 12-2. FLOWCHART. Computer exercise—case study. Head injury—® epidural hematoma.

213

By collecting data from patient records, it is possible to make the CSE as realistic as possible. In all the case studies used, the identity of all the patients is kept confidential.

It may also be necessary to weigh decisions about factors such as the sex, age, and psychosocial status of the patient in the CSE. For example, the effect of head injury on a patient's neurological status has implications for activities of daily living (ADL) as well as psychosocial implications. The next step in developing a CSE is plotting its direction and the courses the patient will take. This may take the form of a flow chart or blueprint.

THE BLUEPRINT

In the example of the head injury CSE, the blueprint consists of a flowchart that shows each component or course of the CSE (See Figure 12–2). The CSE is written from the flow chart. The flow chart may be revised several times while writing the CSE.

The flow chart allows the author to visualize the complicated branching pattern within the program. The branching pattern consists of numerous courses or feedback loops that the learner may enter depending on the type of data or the intervention(s) that are selected.

For example, the CSE on head injury is composed of three courses. The patient initially presents with signs and symptoms of an epidural hematoma. In course I, if the learner assesses the situation correctly and selects the appropriate nursing interventions early on, the epidural hematoma is discovered and evacuated. The patient recovers with some minor complications. In course II, the patient continues to deteriorate and herniates because the signs and symptoms of herniation were not detected by the learner. In course III, the learner detects that herniation is occurring. The epidural hematoma is evaluated and the patient is left with some neurological deficits. After one course is completed, the learner may reenter the program and enter one of the other courses by selecting different choices. Each course offers a different learning situation. The CSE on spinal cord injury is composed of two courses, each of which represents a different patient, both of whom were in the same motor vehicle accident. The learner selects which patient to care for and has the option of reentering the CSE after one course is completed, to care for the other patient. Each patient has sustained a different type of spinal cord injury, one a complete spinal cord injury and the other an incomplete spinal cord injury that can be prevented in the CSE.

WRITING THE CSE

When writing a CSE, one of the most important design considerations is "non-cueing". The problem with many CSEs is that they cue the learner. For example, the learner who is not familiar with the subject matter can deduce answers without learning because the list of choices gives significant clues (Gapanoff et al, 1982). In order to avoid cueing, a generalized list of choices, which appears in the cookbook, is needed. For a given choice, a short feedback message, a more specific list of choices, or another course appears (See Figure 12–3).

This list of generalized choices may be used in more than one CSE. Some questions, however, require an individualized group of choices that may appear only one time in the CSE (See Figure 12–4). A generalized list of choices would be inappropriate in this situation.

It is possible to incorporate new design features in CSE. For the head injury, one of these included the use of the Glasgow Coma Scale (GCS). In this CSE, the learner makes serial assessments of the patient using the coma scale. A graphic display of the coma scale (See Figure 12–5) appears in the CSE. The learner plots out the coma scale and receives feedback on whether they are right or wrong at the end of the CSE. Graphic displays of the patient's intracranial pressure values and measurements of intracranial elastance also appear in the CSE on head injury (See Figure 12–6). Another CSE uses a graphic display of the Denver Developmental Screening Test, in which the patient's progress is plotted out during the CSE. Tables of common laboratory values and tests can also appear throughout the CSE. Any graphic display can be entered into the computer, thus creating infinite possibilities for the CSE.

A common question is, "How long does it take you to write a CSE?" Authoring a CSE can take as little as 6 hours (with a cookbook that is already developed) or as long as 240 hours to complete, including research time for the case studies. The time estimated depends on whether the development of a cookbook is a necessary part of writing the CSE and how complicated the branching pattern of the CSE is. For example, the CSE on spinal cord injury took an estimated 40 hours to write, with a cookbook that was already written. The time for authoring a CSE does not include the time spent "cleaning up" bugs and typing errors in the text once the CSE has been entered into the computer. This could take up to an additional 10 to 20 hours.

When discussing authorship of CSE, it is believed that it would be difficult for anybody to produce computer-based materials by themselves (Chambers and Sprecher, 1980). A team approach has been suggested for developing CSE. It consists of a programmer, an

```
2:00 PM - Joan is admitted to the neurological unit.  As a staff nurse,
what do you need to assess in order to formulate a plan of nursing care?

1.  Circulatory
2.  History
3.  Respiratory
4.  Urinary
5.  Neurological
6.  Lab tests
7.  recap
8.  finished

Enter one number
-->3
Respiratory - resp. 22 regular, lungs clear on ausculation

Enter one number
-->1
Circulatory - 132/78, p-75 regular (supine); 120;72, p-78 (sitting)

Enter one number
-->5
Neurological (choose area(s) below

1.  LOC
2.  motor
3.  pupillary response
4.  sensory
5.  cerebellar
6.  reflexes
7.  all of the above
8.  finished

Enter one or more numbers, separated by commas, then press RETURN
-->7
NEURO-LOC - eyes closed when you walk into her room.  She appears restless
    on the bed.  You call Joan's name to arouse her.  oriented - x3.  She
    is sleepy and opens her eyes after you ask her.
NEURO-motor - 5/5 UE/LE, L arm drifts slightly down and pronates when you ask
    her to hold her arms up.
NEURO-pupillary response - R pupil 5mm, Rx sluggishly to light, L pupil
    3mm Rx briskly to light, EOM intact, nystagmus absent.
NEURO-sensory - intact to V, PP, PS.
NEURO-cerebellar - RAM intact: F-->N, H-->S intact, gait not assessed
NEURO-reflexes - +2 symmetrical, toes--bilateral flexor plantar response

To continue press RETURN-->
2:00 PM - Joan is admitted to the neurological unit.  As a staff nurse,
what do you need to assess in order to formulate a plan of nursing care?

1.  Circulatory
2.  History
3.  Respiratory
4.  Urinary
5.  Neurological
6.  Lab tests
7.  recap
8.  finished

Enter one number
-->6
Lab Data/Diagnostic Tests
1.  fluid and electrolytes
2.  ABG's
3.  finished
Enter one number
-->1
fluid and electrolytes -      Na 142      3.8 K+          125 Glucose
                              Cl 107      23 CO2           15 BUN

    You did this at noon.  Not necessary now.
Enter one number
-->3
```

FIG.12–3. Excerpt from CSE (Note choices and feedback).

```
To continue press RETURN-->_
Post-OP Day #3

    Joan is still on assisted mechanical ventilation and is breathing more
rapidly. ICP was measured at 15 mm Hg.  The following therapies can be
used in the medical management of intracranial hypertension: hyperventilation
(maintain PaCO2 20-25 mm Hg); hyperosmotic agents (mannitol and glycerol),
corticosteroids, lasix, barbituate coma, hypothermia and ventricular drainage.


To continue press RETURN-->_
    Which of the following patient/nurse activities have the potential to
increase ICP?

1.  Turning, moving, up and down in bed and pushing in bed
2.  Decerebrate posturing
3.  Straining during a bowel movement
4.  Conversation about fears, concerns and prognosis about a patient in his
    presence
5.  Head and body positions such as rotating the head, flexing and extending
    the neck and extreme hip flexion
6.  Valsalva maneuver
7.  PEEP (positive end-expiratory pressure ventilation)
8.  Occluded airway
9.  Grouping nursing activities together, so the patient can rest
10. Suctioning the patient between 10 - 15 seconds
11. all of above
Enter one or more numbers, separated by commas, then press RETURN
```

FIG.12–4.   *Excerpts from CSE illustrating individualized group of choices*

instructional designer, and the faculty. This would encourage high-quality programs, would reduce the number of faculty hours to develop CSE, and would increase the number of faculty members developing CSE (Chambers and Sprecher, 1980).

EVALUATION

After the CSE is completed, it can be reviewed by people who have an expertise in the particular area of nursing considered in the CSE, such as patients with head injury or spinal cord injury. Students also use the CSE before it is finalized. Some changes are made in the CSE based on the reviewers' and students' comments. Finally, the CSE can be formally integrated into the curriculum, as occurred with the Nervous System Pathway, at the University of Washington School of Nursing.

Part of the evaluation process can allow the learners to enter their comments directly into the computer at any point of the CSE. A log file of all the comments is kept, and can be reviewed by the author and the programmer. Comments about portions of the CSE that are causing difficulties or that are enjoyable can be entered into the log file. An evaluation form can be given to students to use when they run a CSE. It asks the learner to rate overall design of the CSE, its difficulty, its effectiveness as a teaching tool, the number of hours required to complete it, gaps or incongruities in the CSE, and sugges-

```
 A
 You will now enter your rating of the patient on the Glascow Coma Scale.Would
 you like to review the most recent neurological exam findings first?

 -->n
 What is your patient's coma scale rating at this time?

       Eyes open            Best verbal response         Best motor response

 4  spontaneously       5   oriented                 6   obeys commands
 3  to speech           4   confused                 5   localizes pain
 2  to pain             3   inappropriate            4   flexion-withdrawl
 1  none                2   noncomprehensible        3   abnormal flexion
                        1   none                     2   abnormal extension
                        T   intubated                1   none
 Eyes open ?-->2
 Best verbal response ? (enter number or a 'T')-->4
 Best motor response ?-->4
 Cumulative patient coma scale rating:
          TIME:            ! NOON ! 2 PM ! 3 PM !
    Eyes open
 4  spontaneously         !  *   !      !      !
 3  to speech             !      !  *   !      !
 2  to pain               !      !      !  *   !
 1  none                  !      !      !      !
    Best verbal response
 5  oriented              !  *   !  *   !      !
 4  confused              !      !      !  *   !
 3  inappropriate         !      !      !      !
 2  noncomprehensible     !      !      !      !
 1  none                  !      !      !      !
 T  intubated             !      !      !      !
    Best motor response
 6  obeys commands        !  *   !  *   !      !
 5  localizes pain        !      !      !      !
 4  flexion-withdrawl     !      !      !  *   !
 3  abnormal flexion      !      !      !      !
 2  abnormal extension    !      !      !      !
 1  none                  !      !      !      !

 To continue press RETURN-->


 B

 To continue press RETURN-->
 Cumulative patient coma scale rating:
          TIME:            ! NOON ! 2 PM ! 3 PM ! 10 PM ! Day 5 !
    Eyes open
 4  spontaneously         ! *@  !      !      !       !  *@  !
 3  to speech             !      !  *@  !      !       !      !
 2  to pain               !      !      !  *@  !  *   !      !
 1  none                  !      !      !      !       !      !
    Best verbal response
 5  oriented              ! *@  !  *@  !      !       !      !
 4  confused              !      !      !  *   !       !  @   !
 3  inappropriate         !      !      !  @   !       !      !
 2  noncomprehensible     !      !      !      !       !      !
 1  none                  !      !      !      !       !      !
 T  intubated             !      !      !      !  *@  !  *   !
    Best motor response
 6  obeys commands        ! *@  !  *@  !      !       !  @   !
 5  localizes pain        !      !      !  @   !  @   !      !
 4  flexion-withdrawl     !      !      !  *   !  *   !  *   !
 3  abnormal flexion      !      !      !      !       !      !
 2  abnormal extension    !      !      !      !       !      !
 1  none                  !      !      !      !       !      !
 Comparison of your and author's coma scale ratings:  * = yours,  @ = author's.

 To continue press RETURN-->
 Would you like to see a bibliography?-->n
 You chose  83 correct responses out of  94  scored responses.
 Thank you, Generic Nurse, for participating.
 Would you like to try this program again?-->n
```

FIG.12–5A&B. *Excerpts from CSE (A) Note how student is asked to rate patient on coma scale. (B) Note how coma scale results can be graphically displayed.*

218

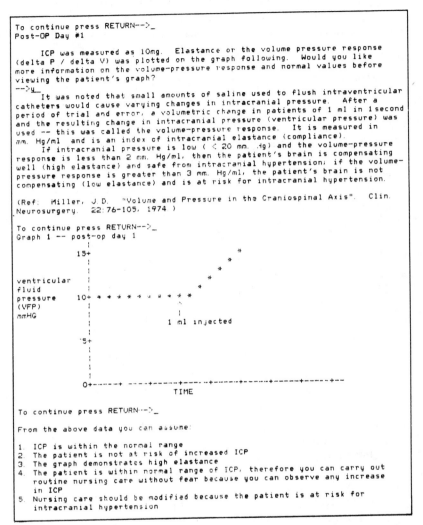

```
To continue press RETURN-->_
Post-OP Day #1

     ICP was measured as 10mg.  Elastance or the volume pressure response
(delta P / delta V) was plotted on the graph following.  Would you like
more information on the volume-pressure response and normal values before
viewing the patient's graph?
-->y_
      It was noted that small amounts of saline used to flush intraventricular
catheters would cause varying changes in intracranial pressure.  After a
period of trial and error, a volumetric change in patients of 1 ml in 1second
and the resulting change in intracranial pressure (ventricular pressure) was
used -- this was called the volume-pressure response.  It is measured in
mm. Hg/ml  and is an index of intracranial elastance (compliance).
      If intracranial pressure is low ( < 20 mm. Hg) and the volume-pressure
response is less than 2 mm. Hg/ml, then the patient's brain is compensating
well (high elastance) and safe from intracranial hypertension; if the volume-
pressure response is greater than 3 mm. Hg/ml, the patient's brain is not
compensating (low elastance) and is at risk for intracranial hypertension.

(Ref:  Miller,  J. D.  "Volume and Pressure in the Craniospinal Axis".  Clin.
Neurosurgery.  22:76-105, 1974 )

To continue press RETURN-->_
Graph 1 -- post-op day 1

           15+                                    *
                                               *
                                            *
ventricular                              *
fluid
pressure   10+  * * * * * * * * * *
(VFP)
mmHG                          
                                1 ml injected

           ˉ5+

            0+------+ ----+-------+-----+------+------+-----+--
                              TIME

To continue press RETURN-->_

From the above data you can assume:

1. ICP is within the normal range
2. The patient is not at risk of increased ICP
3. The graph demonstrates high elastance
4. The patient is within normal range of ICP, therefore you can carry out
   routine nursing care without fear because you can observe any increase
   in ICP
5. Nursing care should be modified because the patient is at risk for
   intracranial hypertension
```

FIG.12–6.   *CSE excerpt shows a graphic display of Intracranial Pressure Measurements.*

tions for future CSE. The form also asks for the learner's area of expertise, so that the difficulty of the CSE can be correlated with their background.

In our experience, all of the students indicated that CSE was an effective teaching tool and wanted to see more developed in other areas. The students' general comments were extremely valuable and helped detect problems or points of disagreement regarding answers. Discussions resulted from this which further facilitated learning.

One of the problems the students may encounter is working with a computer terminal. Most of our students were in their late twenties to early thirties and this was their first exposure to the use of the computer. They were given 10 weeks to do 4 CSEs. Several of the students were frustrated the first time they ran a CSE. They found that if they did not respond exactly as the computer asked them to, they got stuck on a question and could not get out of it. The second time they tried a CSE, they avoided many of the earlier problems because they were familiar with how the terminal worked and the overall design of the CSE. Some of the students did not like the "non-cueing" lists and they were unsure of how much or how little data to ask for. While frustrating to the student, this is a problem one often encounters when collecting data from a patient in the clinical area, thus making CSE more realistic.

To alleviate some of the problems, the students were given a session introducing them to CSE and use of a computer terminal. The goal of this session was to familiarize the student with the technical aspects of working with computers and to reduce any anxiety they might have about them. We discussed such topics as "logging into" the system, getting out of the system, and how to type in comments. A sample of a CSE was also run.

Chambers and Sprecher (1980) concluded that

the use of computer-assisted instruction (CAI)* either improved learning or showed no differences when compared to the traditional classroom approach,

the use of CAI reduced learning time when compared to the regular classroom,

the use of CAI improved student attitudes toward the use of computers in the learning situation, and

the development of CAI coursework following specified guidelines can result in portability and their acceptance and use by other faculty."

USE OF CSE

Throughout this discussion on CSE, we have used the term learner or student to refer to users of CSE. CSE have wide applications in nursing education, including providing problem-solving experiences outside the clinical setting, more efficient use of student and faculty time, and more flexibility in learning. CSE should not be

* Synonymous with CSE in this chapter.

confined to schools of nursing only. With the popular use of micro-computers, CSE would be ideal for use in the hospital by staff nurses, nurse specialists, and nurses in staff development for orientation and inservice. CSE can also be used at home with a portable terminal, further broadening its application. For example, continuing educa-tion credits could be gained at home by completing a CSE in a given specialty area. CSE has enormous potential in nursing.

CONCLUSION

Technology has made new learning experiences possible and CSE in nursing education is such an achievement. CSE offers the learner, whether student, staff nurse, nurse specialist, or educator, opportunities that traditional teaching methods cannot provide. CSE can be run wherever a microcomputer or computer terminal is avail-able. Users of CSE will have a first-hand opportunity to select data, make decisions about patient care and see the consequences of their decisions outside the patient's room. We have entered an exciting age in nursing education that uses technology to develop diagnostic rea-soning and encourages a new type of learning.

BIBLIOGRAPHY

Chambers J, Sprecher J: Computer Assisted Instruction: Current Trends and Critical Issues. Communications of the ACM 23:332–342, 1980

Gaponoff M et al: Medical Simulation: Tutorials, Videodiscs, and Microcom-puters. From Leventhal L (ed): Modeling and Simulation on Microcom-puters. pp. 85–88, La Jolla, Simulation Councils, Inc, 1981

McGuire C: Simulation Technique in Teaching and Testing of Problem Solv-ing Skills. Proceedings of the 46th Annual Meeting of the National Asso-ciation for Research in Science Teaching, March, 1973 (ERIC ED 091 152)

Pearson B: Simulation Techniques for Nursing Education. International Nursing Review 22:144–146, 1975

Pearson B: Evaluation of the Nursing Processes through Visual Motion Me-dia. International Nursing Review 25:119–120, 1978

Pearson B: A Study of the Effects of Teacher Gender on Learning. Image 13:15–17, February, 1981

SECTION FIVE

Diagnostic Reasoning in Nursing: Some Professional Implications

Doris L. Carnevali

CHAPTER THIRTEEN

Strategies for Self-Monitoring of Diagnostic Reasoning Behaviors: Pathway to Professional Growth

Doris L. Carnevali

Diagnostic reasoning is a very personal activity. Others can observe the overt behavior and the products (verbal or written statements of the data base, problems ruled out, impressions and diagnoses), but it is the diagnostician who can engage in self-observation of the critical thinking that produces these behaviors and products. Admittedly, such self-monitoring is limited by one's knowledge base and experience. It may also be influenced by some blind spots and biases. Still, self-analysis is a useful tool in gaining greater awareness and skill in diagnostic reasoning.

A series of questions or observational guidelines may help the reader attain a greater awareness of current practices being used in diagnostic reasoning. Two strategies are possible. One involves concurrent observation as the diagnostic reasoning is occurring. The other involves working backwards from action to diagnosis to the data from which the diagnosis derived; it is a retrospective approach.

CONCURRENT OBSERVATION OF ONE'S DIAGNOSTIC REASONING PROCESS

Concurrent self-observation of one's diagnostic reasoning process might be likened to having a "watchbird" perched on one's

225

shoulder serving as an outside observer to what one is doing. If this technique is used, the following questions and observational guides may be useful.

- □ What are the risk areas, problem areas, or priorities of attention that tend to come to my mind, because of my specialty or background, just before my initial encounter with a patient?
- □ What pre-encounter patient data do I value,? seek,? use to structure the initial observations,? narrow the data search field?
- □ What aspects of the patient data field do I tend to notice first?
- □ How do I structure my initial behavior in relationship to the patient to shape the direction of data he provides?
- □ Is there a pattern to my early data collection? What is it?
- □ How soon in the data collecting process do I find myself generating diagnostic possibilities?
- □ How many possible diagnoses do I tend to activate in this first retrieval?
- □ Is there any hierarchical arrangement to them such as general problem areas and sub problem possibilities that are more specific, e.g., communication—problem in speaking, problem understanding English?
- □ Do I tend to generate competing diagnoses,? e.g., anger in grief vs anger in frustration or immobilization leading to sensory deprivation vs sensory deprivation leading to immobilization?
- □ How do the diagnostic hypotheses I bring to mind affect my subsequent data collection?

> Do I gather data associated with the particular diagnostic hypothesis?
>
> Do I continue to gather data according to an instrument or usual system, but notice/cluster cues related to the diagnostic hypotheses?
>
> Do I combine both strategies?

- □ What do I do with disconfirming data? How am I storing data that may not fit current diagnostic areas, but may be important—possibly in treatment decisions?

☐ Do I gather data on strengths in patterns of daily living, internal/external resources as well as deficits?

☐ What data am I using to explicitly rule out problem areas?

☐ How do I go about evaluating the goodness of fit between the patient's presenting data and the profile of risk factors, and antecedent events and manifestations associated with the diagnostic hypotheses I am testing?

☐ How precisely does my final diagnostic statement incorporate the patient's presenting situation as distinguishable from that of other patients whose problems in daily living-health status fall within this general problem area?

☐ Am I predicting the risks of future problems based on patient data and my professional knowledge of new demands in daily living or further diminution of internal–external resources?

It may be possible to engage in self-analysis in only one or two areas in the beginning, and gradually work through the entire series. As one becomes familiar with each aspect and comfortable with it, then it may be possible to do self-analysis using the entire diagnostic reasoning process on one case. It is also possible to assess trends and patterns in one's diagnostic reasoning behavior and to observe changes over time.

RETROSPECTIVE ANALYSIS OF ONE'S DIAGNOSTIC REASONING

A second strategy for discovering one's diagnostic reasoning behavior is that of working backwards. In this technique, one begins with the nursing action being engaged in and thinks backward through the implicit diagnosis that served as the impetus for that action and finally back to the data that actually were used to arrive at the diagnosis. The following questions may serve to guide this type of analysis.

☐ What nursing activities am I undertaking with this patient or family? Am I carrying them out in a particular manner?

- □ How am I doing these activities differently with this patient or family than with others having a similar problem?

- □ What areas of daily living–developmental tasks are involved? What aspects of health status affect these tasks? Are external resources involved? If so, what is their status that has affected the nursing actions being undertaken?

- □ Why was the action or skills of a nurse required in this situation,? *i.e.*, Why can't the patient/family deal with this for themselves?

- □ What cues in manifestations (signs or symptoms of inadequacy in managing health-related daily living) or risk factors did I notice as being presented by this patient, family or their environment, that could have led me to discern the problem area in which my action is being taken?

- □ How did my clinical specialty, my work setting, usual clientele, or previous experiences influence what I was prepared to notice and diagnose with this patient or family?

The retrospective approach tends to be somewhat less refined and detailed than the concurrent self-analysis. Perhaps it serves best as an initial strategy for those who are least comfortable with the diagnostic reasoning concept. As comfort and confidence develop, the retrospective approach can be replaced with the introduction and gradually increasing use of the watchbird—concurrent self analysis approach.

SUMMARY

Either of these strategies can be useful to increase one's consciousness of the use of the elements of the diagnostic reasoning process. The reader can determine which serves as the better starting point. Later, each may be used, however the reader is able and willing, for the advancement of skill in diagnostic reasoning. One may concentrate on a particular area for a time and then move on to another component or look at patterns and trends. By whatever approach, the goal is to gain the capability to become more conscious of the process used in one's diagnostic reasoning in order to critique it and hone it to greater sharpness.

CHAPTER FOURTEEN

Development of Diagnostic Reasoning Skills: Implications for Nursing Practice, Education, Management, Nursing Literature, and Research

Doris L. Carnevali

The ultimate beneficiary of well-developed nursing diagnostic skills is the clientele. However, to make these skills consistently available to nursing's clientele (given the current state of the art), some concerted effort is going to be required of nurses in almost all arenas of nursing today. It will include students, practicing clinicians, nursing-care managers, educators, as well as the authors of nursing text books, articles, and nursing researchers.

NURSING STUDENTS AND CLINICIANS

The current challenge to students and clinicians alike is two fold:

☐ development of the knowledge base for diagnosis and expertise in diagnostic reasoning in the *nursing domain,* and
☐ integration of diagnostic reasoning into nursing practice on a consistent routine basis.

229

Diagnostic expertise is never fully achieved. There are always areas and directions for growth, not only for the novice, but for the experienced diagnostician. To engage in this ongoing development, the student or the expert needs to:

- recognize the direction that increasing expertise must take,*

- recognize the need to store experience, not only in episodic memory, but to integrate it into the appropriate diagnostic packets in semantic long-term memory as well,

- organize and cross-reference new knowledge as it is stored, so that it is in a form for efficient retrieval for differential diagnosis, and

- maintain an awareness of the pitfalls associated with each stage of diagnostic development in order to do as much prevention as possible.

In the beginning, growth is obvious to the novice diagnostician. As a nurse becomes increasingly familiar with the process and the diagnostic tasks, the challenge becomes one of the maintaining freshness in one's perspective and enhancing consciously one's diagnostic effectiveness. Experts can always further refurbish and reorganize their diagnostic concepts for greater clinical efficiency. New cross referencing can be established, based on new clinical experiences and understandings. Larger concepts can be developed to encompass and tie together the commonalities of smaller ones—again making retrieval easier and minimizing the space in short-term memory by building the potential for bigger "chunks". For novice and expert alike, the hallmark of professional diagnostic competence is continuing growth and freshness in the diagnostic realm.

The second challenge to the practicing student or clinician is to find realistic strategies for engaging in diagnostic reasoning in one's nursing practice on a consistent, routine basis, given the roles and functions that prevail in the clinical setting. Case loads are heavy. Assignments are unpredictable. Delegated medical functions have a tradition of assuming highest importance and the biomedical focus has consistent preeminence. The nursing perspective is not particularly valued, perhaps not even recognized. Underprepared colleagues feel distressed either by the diagnostic reasoning of another nurse, or by the concommitant threat that they also may be required to engage in this form of critical thinking. Any one or a combination

---

* See Chapter 13 for Self-monitoring strategies

of these conditions make it difficult to engage in nursing-oriented diagnostic reasoning activities. Still, the mind is quick and capable of functioning under a variety of conditions. If both diagnostic reasoning and the nursing domain are valued, ways have been found to function.

NURSING CARE MANAGERS

Mid level nursing care managers (head nurses, care coordinators, and others), have under their supervision nurses with varying degrees of diagnostic experience and skill. As care managers, they have two kinds of responsibilities associated with expertise in diagnostic reasoning:

☐ to assure that patients and their families are adequately and accurately diagnosed in the nursing domain as a basis for their nursing treatment, and

☐ to contribute to the professional development of the nursing diagnosticians under their supervision.

Quality Control in Nursing Diagnosing

Each of the administrative responsibilities—quality control of nursing diagnostic effectiveness and staff development—requires the mid-level nursing managers to be knowledgeable about diagnostic tasks, factors, and skills. While the core of diagnostic reasoning remains constant across diagnostic tasks, the diagnostic tasks themselves differ as does the needed knowledge base. Even the small sample of diagnostic areas illustrated in Section Three gives evidence of both the commonality and variability of diagnostic tasks in differing settings and clientele. Head nurses, clinical coordinators, and supervisors in institutional and community settings need to be highly conscious of the nature and range of diagnostic tasks and challenges their nurses are encountering.

A second area of information care managers need in order to exercise quality control of nursing diagnosis is related to the status of diagnostic expertise of the registered nurse staff. Mere longevity in the profession is no sure measure of the stage of development in the diagnostic reasoning process, particularly given the lack of attention that has been paid to fostering nursing diagnostic skill in both basic nursing programs and continuing education offerings. Thus, just as patients are assessed and diagnosed by their nurses, so practicing nurses need to be assessed to determine their stage of development in diagnostic reasoning by those responsible for the quality of nursing care in that segment of the health-care system. While the behaviors described in Table 3–1 are still tentative and not fully tested, they can be used as some form of an observational guideline to arrive at ball-park judgments about the levels of diagnostic ability for diagnosis of the clientele. These data on nurse diagnostic ability can be used as one variable in assigning client assessments or primary nurse case loads and to suggest where backup or followup may be desirable. Both the quality of nursing diagnosis available to the patient and growth-producing opportunities are variables that the nursing care manager may consider in making assignments.

Staff Development

The education and training of physicians gives much more time and critical attention to their diagnostic reasoning skills. Further, the beginning diagnostic skills of new physicians is honed in progressive complexity and accountability, associated with patient care assignments in their residences. By contrast, because diagnostic reasoning has been less rigorously developed during initial training and education in nursing, staff development in this area often must be quite basic. Staff development programs to further develop diagnostic reasoning skills can take many forms:

☐ Pairing clinicians over a period of time to critique and encourage each other's diagnostic efforts. Changing those pairings periodically to provide fresh perspectives;

☐ Use of patient conferences to work on particularly difficult diagnostic problems or to develop diagnostic concepts that have heavy use with a clientele;

☐ Grand rounds that present patients from a nursing perspective followed by further analysis and critique;

☐ Videotaped vignettes to compare individual staff member's diagnostic strategies and judgments;

☐ Seminars on particular diagnostic concepts and their use with a range of health problems, clientele or settings;

☐ Seminars on the differing use of biomedical data in medical and nursing perspectives;

☐ Collection of journal articles from both nursing and medical journals or Xeroxed copies of book chapters that discuss the diagnostic reasoning process being added to the nursing library. Reports and discussions of ideas and their application to the clientele and the nursing perspective;

☐ Group discussions to develop explicit expectations and norms for inclusion of nursing diagnoses and treatment plans, as well as the biomedical, in communication about patients;

☐ Setting of expectations that clinicians with greater diagnostic expertise will serve as role models on the process and the product, as well as the give and take of critiquing;

☐ Seminars to explore the tangible values associated with explicitly engaging in diagnostic reasoning from a nursing perspective.

Probably the most effective staff development is associated with the multiple, client-oriented incidents occurring daily where diagnostic reasoning occurs. It is here that the nursing care manager can demonstrate that it is required and valued. It is here that the diagnostic reasoning activities can be questioned, further developed, speeded up, and rewarded. The little learnings, day-in, day-out, the new possibilities seen, the mistakes, the successes—all these can be used by the astute care managers to increase the diagnostic reasoning expertise of their staff.

NURSE EDUCATORS

Teachers in nursing have a special obligation to fully assimilate and integrate the knowledge and skills of the diagnostic reasoning process so that these in turn can influence all the elements of their teaching.

From the earliest nursing courses, students should be helped to recognize explicitly why and how nursing knowledge and experience is organized and stored systematically for diagnostic purposes. With factual knowledge, students need to see the importance of storing clear, sharp recognition features of both risk factors and manifestations associated with phenomena in the nursing domain (this storage process is identified with future recognition tasks). Students need to learn early and explicitly the risks of making inferences primarily on the basis of experience alone. Then, they need to learn how to analyze their experiences in order to link them with related diagnostic concepts they have stored in semantic long-term memory.

Students, for their own self development in gaining diagnostic reasoning skill need to know the *kinds of activities* they must deliberately and consciously engage in, on their own:

☐ the acquisition and systematic storage of knowledge from classes, reading, and the integration of retrospectively analyzed clinical experiences, and

☐ the actual critical practice of applying the stored knowledge in the analysis of presenting clinical situations.

Each of these skill areas is interdependent, *but* each is learned in differing modes of practice. Thus, education for diagnostic expertise includes critiqued purposeful practice of both components. These are skills and patterns of professional practice the students can only gain for themselves. The strategies, modelling, and opportunities can be offered, but the students can achieve expertise only by the quality and extensiveness of their own endeavors.

On the other hand, nursing faculty members have multifaceted and demanding responsibilities in teaching and modelling the nature of the diagnostic reasoning process as a *particular* problem-solving approach used in the clinical practice of nursing. This includes providing learning experiences on:

the nursing domain in relationship to the domains of other health-care disciplines—the commonalities, overlaps and differences, the distinguishing features in the perspectives of each,

system(s) for organizing and storing semantic and experiental knowledge for diagnostic purposes—both nursing and biomedical,

techniques for making cross-linkages between related phenomena and diagnostic concepts to develop differential diagnosing skills,

skills of application of the diagnostic reasoning process to the same presenting situation from both the nursing and biomedical domains,

discipline-specific vocabulary and recording systems as well as the behavior required in presenting diagnostic reasoning and clinical judgements for the greater effectiveness,

implications of co-professional role relationships in the

diagnostic and prescriptive areas of professional
practice, and

strategies for gaining credibility and influence for
nursing diagnostic reasoning, diagnoses, and
treatment plans in multidisciplinary practice.

Some of these tasks involve the use of a consistent *system* in which
"factual" content is presented, so that the same organizational out-
line is used for nursing and biomedical diagnostic concepts. (See Figure 14–1 for a sample format.) Such a format can be used to structure
the kind of information, the headings used, and the sequence of
presentation. Linkages between nursing diagnostic concepts can be a
part of the information-giving behavior in both nursing-to-nursing,
nursing-to-biomedical and biomedical-to-nursing concepts. Modelling this cross-linking is important, not only in the presentation of
theory but in the clinical situation.

Some other learning tasks involve clinical assignments and critiqued practice that includes explicit identification of pre-encounter
factors and data, entry to the data field, hypothesis generation, testing, and the actual identification of the diagnosis. Attention also
needs to be given to the use of disconfirming data and data on
strengths noted in daily living patterns, internal resources, and external resources. Again the differences in use of patient data from the
biomedical and nursing diagnostic perspective needs to be differentiated explicitly.

Other learning about the diagnostic reasoning process—valuing
it and learning the associated role behaviors—are more likely to be
assimilated from seeing faculty and staff consistently role model the
expertise and the associated vulnerability and accountability, the
sharing aloud of their thinking patterns and rationale in a given situation, and the actual encouragement of student critique. The strategies for getting diagnostic reasoning from the nursing perspective
into the system as an influential element in the patient's health-care
plan, and fitting the nurse's diagnostic behavior realistically into the
health-care system, probably takes an honest and consistent amalga-
mation of the clinical faculty member with other role models in the
health-care system where the care is being delivered.

Given the state of the art of diagnostic reasoning in nursing and
the limited level of acceptance of a distinct domain for nursing diagnosis, what is being proposed here is no mean task. However, if a
critical mass of nurses, who are capable of holding their own, diagnostically, in the health-care system, is to emerge, it is a critical task
for nursing educators.

Title	DIAGNOSTIC CONCEPT TITLE
Overall definition	General description of the category of problem or phenomenon
Etiology	Antecedent or current events, factors in environment, changes or predicted changes in internal or external resources that precede the occurrence of the problem
Risk factors	Characteristic features of persons who have a higher probability of having this situation; conditions, situations or time periods when there is increased risk of occurrence
Dynamics	Underlying mechanisms of the problem—what is occurring, how it is being made to happen, what variables are involved
Manifestations (signs and symptoms)	Patterns of cues (subjective/objective) that together present the profile needed to assign the phenomenon/problem to this diagnostic category
Differential diagnosis	Other diagnostic concepts that need to be considered as a basis for making the most precise classification and the best basis for treatment
Complications	Additional undesired sequelae or side-effects that can occur secondary to the primary problem
Prognosis	Predicted direction, duration, and range of outcomes, together with the factors that contribute to them and thus enable prediction
Prevention and management	Actions predicted to most effectively prevent the problem or enable effective management of daily living (general guidelines that must be individualized on the basis of presenting data in the given situation)
Evaluation	Areas of data collection on the client and his situation that will indicate the nature of response to treatment plus criteria for interpreting the data in terms of improvement or lack of it

FIG.14–1. *Format for organizing and storing nursing knowledge to expedite diagnostic reasoning (Adapted from Carnevali D: Nursing Care Planning: Diagnosis and Management, 3rd ed., Philadelphia, J.B. Lippincott, 1983)*

NURSING AUTHORS

Those who write for nursing, particularly those who write textbooks for nursing students, have major responsibilities for organizing topics and content in such a format as to expedite sound diagnostic reasoning patterns in nursing (see Fig. 14–1). This raises several issues.

One issue is the appropriate separation of, and parity for, nursing diagnostic concepts in relationship to biomedical diagnostic concepts, without losing the necessary cross-linkages between them. The day is past when textbooks introduce nursing aspects of patient care as what the nurse does—after the medical diagnosis and treatment plan has been fully addressed. Nursing is no longer just a subset to medical treatment. Reality dictates that nurses will continue to engage in delegated medical functions of both diagnosis and treatment. They must also understand the dynamics of pathology—pathophysiology and psychopathology—as a basis for many nursing diagnoses and plans of treatment. The challenge to nursing authors comes then in giving each domain its proper place and in explicitly demonstrating the linkages between knowledge in each one. To take an example in another field, chemists and chemistry texts use both mathematics and physics content extensively, yet in chemistry texts, they are mere tools to expedite the understanding of the discipline of chemistry. Just so, nursing texts need to give adequate attention to the knowledge of associated disciplines, but to cast this knowledge always within the framework of the nursing discipline. Such thinking and writing, such organization of textbook content, will require some fresh thinking, which is difficult (as writers in this book will readily testify). Yet the models are there in other disciplines' textbooks. Nursing authors simply need to adapt these patterns to the nursing domain and the dual type of focus that is required of nurses.

NURSING RESEARCHERS

One of the major limitations to rigor in diagnostic reasoning and rational nursing treatment is the lack of a researched block of knowledge comparable to pathophysiology in the biomedical domain. Nursing research is clearly needed along the following lines:

- □ to identify and describe daily living/developmental task-health ↔ status-problem areas,
- □ to describe characteristics (risk factors, manifestations) associated with each problem area,
- □ to describe antecedent events associated with particular phenomena in these problem areas,

- [ ] to define predominant distinguishing characteristics—patterns of cues and risk factors that are more closely associated with one diagnosis than with another
- [ ] to describe the underlying mechanisms that are producing the phenomena—the variables involved and how they interact,
- [ ] to describe potential trajectories and outcomes together with the variables that are predictors of these prognostic options in the daily living/developmental task and health-status perspective,
- [ ] to describe complications associated with the phenomena and with various forms of nursing treatment, and
- [ ] to generate and test nursing treatment regimens so as to understand why and how they can affect the phenomena being treated.

Examples of such research are becoming increasingly visible in the nursing literature. More than two decades ago, the phenomenon of sensory deprivation in patients undergoing eye surgery was observed and described. Later, the category of sensory perceptual alteration was extended with observations of postcardiotomy patients demonstrating similar cues. In another area, nursing assessment of the possibility of domestic violence stems from studies of risk factors and cues related to battering. Diagnostic categories related to maternal attachment will surely evolve from the multiple studies now ongoing that focus on risk factors and cues related to adoption of maternal roles. Only as our descriptive research is developed and health status–daily-living phenomena are understood, can risk factors be delineated for preventive strategies. Only then can precise differential diagnoses be made possible and rational treatment options be generated and tested.

SUMMARY

Movement toward a more diagnostically and prescriptively oriented nursing practice has implications for students, clinicians, nursing care managers, teachers, writers, and researchers. As nurses in each of these nursing fields acknowledge and integrate into their practice the distinct domain for nursing and the diagnostic reasoning process, nursing will progress.

INDEX

Note: Page numbers in *italics* indicate page numbers; those followed by *t* indicate tables; those followed by *n* indicate footnotes.

Abdominal tumors, 108
Activities of daily living. *See* Daily
  living, activities of
Algorithms, 206

Bayes' theorem, 200
Biological status, normal age-related,
  6–7
Bone tumors, 108
  metastatic, patient log in, 118–119,
  129–130
Brain herniation, in critical care patient, 166
Brain tumors, 108
Breast cancer, patient log in, 118–119,
  129–130

Cancer
  abdominal, 108
  advanced
    biomedical vs. nursing prognoses
    in, 126
    home nursing in
      demands of daily living in, 117
      diagnosis-directed data search
      in, 121–125
      diagnostic categories in, 120
      early areas of data collection in,
      111–113
      entry to data field in, 110–120
      environmental supports and
      barriers in, 116
      face-to-face encounters in, 111
      family's knowledge of patient's
      health status in, 115
      fatigue assessment in, 123–125
      health care providers in, 115–
      116
      hypothesis activation in, 120–
      121
      hypothesis testing in, 125
      initial assessment in, 110–120
      closure of, 119–120
      pain assessment in, 121–123
      patient goals in, early data
      collection for, 111–112
      patient-kept log in, 118–119,
      129t–130t

patient's knowledge of disease
  in, 113
patient's pets in, 115
patient's physical status in, 116–
  117
patient's role in ongoing assessment in, 117–118
patient's support systems in,
  114
patterns of activities in, 117
phone contacts in, 110–111
pre-encounter patient data in,
  108–109
pre-entry factors in, 107–110
prognostic variables in, 126–128
setting-based factors in, 109–110
bone, 108
  metastatic, patient log in, 118–119,
  129–130
brain, 108
breast, patient log in, 118–119, 129–
  130
types of, and daily living, 108
Categories
  diagnostic
    activation of, 75–76
    in home cancer nursing, 120
Chronic renal failure. *See* Renal disease, end-stage
Chunking, by hypothesis activation, 89
Chunks of information
  capacity of short-term memory for,
  43
  defined, 43
Classification system. *See also* Taxono-
  my(ies)
  constructability of, 186
  desirable characteristics of, 182–186
  disjoint, 183, 184t
  exhaustive, 183
  natural, 182
  parallel levels of abstraction in, 185,
  185t
  principle of ordering of, 184–185
  relevant, 182–183
  usefulness of, 185–186
Communication, as internal resource,
  19

239